A DOCTOR'S ODYSSEY

A DOCTOR'S ODYSSEY

Nessan McCann, MD

The Book Guild Ltd
Sussex, England

This book is sold subject to the condition that it shall not, by way of trade or otherwise, be lent, re-sold, hired out, photocopied or held in any retrieval system or otherwise circulated without the publisher's prior consent in any form of binding or cover other than that in which this is published and without a similar condition including this condition being imposed on the subsequent purchaser.

The Book Guild Ltd,
25 High Street,
Lewes, Sussex

First published 1999
© Nessan McCann 1999

Set in Times
Typesetting by IML Typographers, Chester
Printed in Great Britain by
Bookcraft (Bath) Ltd, Avon

A catalogue record for this book is
available from the British Library

ISBN 1 85776 455 2

This book is dedicated to Betty, my wife, with all my love.

CONTENTS

1	First Practice – Northern Ireland (1949–52)	1
2	Married Bliss and Addiction	23
3	Second Practice – Northern Ireland (1953–59)	33
4	Gathering Storms	53
5	Flight to Freedom	58
6	Life in Avej	70
7	Where Next?	90
8	Winter and a Decision	98
9	A Lengthy Divorce in Reno	107
10	Back to England	118
11	Ghana, West Africa	126
12	Sierra Leone, West Africa	134
13	United States and Canada	141
14	Yale, New Haven	152
15	Private Practice – Florida	166
16	Washington, DC	174
17	Prison Doctor	177
18	Postponing Retirement	184

PREFACE

This is not the story of a successful doctor, brilliant diagnoses or miraculous cures. It has been said by a wise doctor, and I agree, that 'God cures the patient, though the doctor collects the fee.'

A doctor leads two lives; one deals with patients and their problems and the other deals with his own life and problems. Though intermingled I have tried to separate the two, or at least emphasize the problems encountered in my personal life, because that is what friends and acquaintances find most interesting and ask me to relate.

None of this would have been possible without the support and encouragement of one woman, my wife Betty. She came into my life in my darkest hour, and her faith and belief in my potential lent impetus to my escape from disaster. Her extreme capability and my own optimism have prevailed down through the years leading to the story which you are about to read. I hope you enjoy it as much as I have in recalling and writing it.

St Augustine, Florida
July, 1998

1

First Practice – Northern Ireland (1949–52)

In the two years before December 1959 Vincent McGovern, otherwise known as the 'Bush', had become my best friend, so he volunteered to drive me to Dublin airport four days before Christmas. I was on my way to Iran to spend two years as a physician on a road-building project operated by The Plan Organization. My wife, son aged seven, and daughter aged five, came along and our party was sorrowful but we were consoled by the fact that it would be only a two-year separation.

How wrong we were. I would never again see my wife and I would see my children only three times for brief visits in the next 37 years.

I had been very successful in two practices, one in County Tyrone and one in County Fermanagh during the previous eight years – if success meant treating patients successfully, accumulating an increasing patient panel and being popular in the community. However, viewed from the standpoint of financial success and family happiness, the story was quite different, beginning eight years earlier. Although I loved the children and they loved me, the house was divided against itself.

Having graduated at the National University of Ireland, Dublin, in 1949 six months after my girlfriend of six years, I had many offers of locum tenens positions. My father, a general practitioner in an enormous practice in Dublin, came down with acute lumbago and asked me to help him out. I sent my girlfriend to fill a lucrative locum tenens position in Northern Ireland while I helped my father. I enjoyed working with my father and in the month I worked with him he taught me many useful lessons which have lasted me all my career.

When my girlfriend came back from her locum she had become engaged to her employer, a successful wealthy established practitioner who lived with his mother.

After my father recovered his independence I accepted a locum in Fintona, Northern Ireland, covering a doctor who was going to the United States for three months' vacation. I would be working with his father, an elderly practitioner, while his son was in America.

The British National Health Service had been established in 1948 and on the British mainland a practice could not be set up without approval of the government. In Northern Ireland, however, although it was part of the United Kingdom, it was still legal to establish a practice and then to notify the government. The older doctor in the practice where I did the locum, a Dr Frank Bradley, advised me to set up a practice in Gortin, 20 miles away, where his cousin was getting on in years and probably going to retire. We went to see him and he said he had no objection to my setting up a practice in the small town, which was surrounded by mountains in County Tyrone.

After a brief return to Dublin I said goodbye to my parents and returned to set up my practice in Gortin.

Fintona is situated in the south-west of County Tyrone and was then a fairly large town with a population of approximately 3,000 with a wide social range from the very poor to the moderately rich and surrounded by good farming land and farmers who were fairly comfortably well off.

Before the British National Health Service started in 1948, the old panel practice was run by Dr Frank Bradley. There was a doctor's surgery separate from where he lived. This was in a side street at the upper end of the town, which was built on the side of a hill and it was a lock-up. (He saw private patients in a more comfortable surgery attached to his home, where there was heating in the waiting room and the consulting room.) It was kept locked after consultation hours ended. At the inception of the NHS the dispensary and consulting room in town was closed, locked and left. It was from this that I stocked my dispensary when I started my practice in Gortin.

When I first arrived in Fintona in January 1950, I had driven from Dublin with the local Fintona dentist, who was recovering from surgery in Dublin. He had a new car and I had the pleasure of driving him to Fintona.

I had obtained the locum tenens job for three months through my brother Kevin, who had met Dr Seamus Bradley during a post-graduate course in public health in Dublin. Dr Seamus was going to America for at least three months and it was rumoured that he might go and stay there permanently, if I were to believe his mother when I was doing the locum. Before I left for Dublin at the end of my locum, she confided in me that 'Daddy' (Dr Frank) was going to offer me an invitation to join the practice when he was ready to retire – a pipe dream with no truth.

Their house was one of the largest in the area and it was built on a hill overlooking the town on about an acre of ground with a two-car garage. There was a tennis court with wide lawns between the house and the highway. It was a large home with about five bedrooms and an enormous master bedroom, under which there was a spacious sitting room. Dr Frank Bradley had overseen the building of it and spared no expense. Even though I had spent most of my youth in a three-storey six-bedroom house in Dublin, I was nevertheless very impressed by the Bradley home which by comparison with mine was very modern.

Dr Seamus was a bachelor; one of his sisters, Marie, lived in the home and managed everything from the maid to the meals. Her mother, Mrs Bradley, seemed to be a semi-invalid and could do nothing but get up in the morning, sit in the sitting room, go to her meals and go to bed. She smoked heavily when she could get somebody to give her cigarettes. When I arrived I had given up cigarettes for the New Year but the old lady persuaded me to start smoking again, and she was never short of cigarettes while I was there. She was a dreamer and related stories of her youth and her earlier life in Fintona, during which apparently she did little other than play golf, tennis and go shopping for clothes.

The practice was divided between Dr Bradley senior, and Dr Bradley junior. The senior had the greater part of the practice, earning two-thirds of the annual income. Two-thirds of the patients were registered in his name and one-third in the name of his son Seamus. This was fair, because Dr Bradley senior took responsibility for the practice expenses. He paid for the upkeep of the house and consulting rooms as well as the cars. He had taken his son in as an assistant and later had made him a one-third partner.

When I arrived Seamus showed me how to run the practice, how to deal with patients and how to run the anaesthetic apparatus. He explained the system for filling government forms for delivering babies, anaesthetics for the dentist etc. He stayed with me for a few days and also explained that if any patients came in, I was to ask them to bring their medical cards. These were to be kept in the office until he came back and he would then change them into his name. The reason for this, he said, was that if anything happened to his father, if he died suddenly, it would be very complicated to get the practice transferred to Seamus's name at short notice. I did not think it was part of my job to do this and at no stage during the locum did I follow this procedure.

After Seamus left for the United States I got to know Dr Bradley senior much better and he was a wonderful man and doctor. A man of few words but with a very subtle sense of humour. He had spent the first part of his medical career in South Africa and had some interesting stories to tell of his young medical career there; and other tales of his youth in County Derry, where he was born and grew up. He rarely did house calls which were all left to me, but he was readily available to see patients at all hours of the day in the consulting room. At the evening surgery, I saw the patients. Dr Bradley did the morning surgery.

Dr Frank was an excellent obstetrician and anaesthetist. On a few difficult deliveries he accompanied me and could give all types of anaesthetics, chloroform being one of them although it was then becoming unpopular. It was dangerous in inexperienced hands but I never saw him the slightest bit anxious. He was always calm and comforting to the patients in spite of his advancing years. The new National Health Service made it mandatory to retire at 65 but physicians who were in practice before the inception of the NHS could stay on indefinitely.

When Dr Seamus returned from the United States I went back

to Dublin and made plans to open my practice in Gortin. Two weeks later I returned to hang up my shingle.

I rented two rooms, one as a surgery and one as a bedroom, in the house of the local garage repair man, and he and his wife and children immediately became my first patients. I opened an outlying dispensary, or satellite office, out in the mountains at the borders of Tyrone and Derry and patients gradually began to join my panel. However, I survived on patients who were not members of my panel but who were willing to pay cash until such time they decided to take their cards from whatever doctor they were registered with and change them over to my panel.

My mother had given me £500 in cash to get me over my initial period and to help me to get a car. That was a lot of money in those days. With my advent, the older doctor in Gortin got very active and suddenly was available around the clock on short notice to do house calls and deliveries to the extent that my arrival was considered to be a miracle, rejuvenating the old man and giving him new life!

Using the government Formulary, I was able to dispense medication with few problems. I learned the hard way that there is a difference between tinct belladonna and extract belladonna. The extract is ten times stronger than the tincture. One day I made up a concoction and put in the extract instead of the tincture unintentionally. The following day the patient's husband called me to come and see his wife, so I went to the school (they were both schoolteachers). The lady had been taking my medicine. She looked strange and had been acting strangely. She had apparently offered to make a pot of tea for the parish priest when he came to visit the school earlier that day. She put the tea in a cup and put the cup on top of the stove, splitting it; and that was only one of the many strange things she did. Her dilated pupils were my clue to what was wrong. I told her husband that the medication was a little too strong and I would bring in another bottle for her. When I got back the following day she was normal and naturally I did not tell her that I had almost poisoned her. On my first visit I had of course confiscated the first bottle. Hence her recovery.

The son of the lady in whose house I ran the outlying dispensary (satellite office) had a son aged 17. Every time I came to the dispensary he had a bunch of transfer cards from neighbours around the area. It was not until a year later that I discovered he was canvassing the patients of the old doctor in town. This was a highly irregular procedure and could have got me into a lot of trouble. When I found out what he was doing I had him discontinue it and I apologized to the old doctor. The latter was quite forgiving and laughed, pointing out that his pension when he retired would depend on the number of patients on his panel.

The used car which I had bought in Belfast, from a man I discovered later to be an infamous car dealer, gave me many problems. The first one was on the day I bought it when it blew a hole in the cylinder head. The garage to which it was towed told me that there had been a previous hole which had been welded to keep it going long enough to sell the car. Buying a new cylinder head and staying the night in a hotel sliced further into my mother's £500. The garage repair man with whom I was lodging helped me to repair many of the other problems I had and taught me how to do my own repairs, and he did not charge me for what he had done. The car was a Sunbeam Talbot coupé and even when the top was up it was very cold. There were no car heaters in those days. With all these problems I tried to sell it but hardly could have given it away.

A friend who ran a taxi company was going to London to buy a taxi. He suggested that I go with him and we would drive to the boat and then from Holyhead to London and there he would get me a customer. It was a very enjoyable trip. He had a sister in London who put us up and he ended up trading my car for his new taxi. We drove back in the taxi and on his suggestion I bought a motorcycle to keep me going until I could get a new car. New cars were difficult to obtain but a doctor could get one with a sufficiently sad story. Mine was a sad one and I went to the Ministry and eventually got a new Morris Minor. This was the first new car ever to be seen in Gortin in ten years – or since before the war.

With the help of a very kind bank manager in Omagh to whom I had been introduced by old Mrs Bradley, I was surviving on an overdraft. The practice was gradually improving and I became friendly with a doctor in another town 14 miles away called Carrickmore. He was well established and extremely kind and generous and I covered his practice when he was away. He raced greyhounds, so he frequently went away to a race meeting or to race his greyhounds in Belfast. He reciprocated for me when I went on vacation, which was not often. I did, however, get to Dublin to see my parents every few months.

The practice did not flourish but it was growing steadily, as was my overdraft at the bank, but the kind manager was very patient and encouraged me to continue with the practice and not give up.

While I was the locum for the Doctors Bradley, Dr Frank's other daughter Gloria came home for weekends and we began to date.

I then succeeded in getting a small house in Gortin. The house was so small that the downstairs consisted of a kitchen, living room and parlour. The parlour became a consulting room. There was no pharmacist in the town so I had to dispense medications. Upstairs there was an enormous bathroom so I had that converted into a pharmacy. There was no need to lock it as the only people who went upstairs were myself and, later, my wife. Dr Bradley senior had been a dispensing doctor before the NHS system began in 1948 and he had a full complement of pharmaceuticals. He gave me enough medications to keep me making cough mixtures, stomach mixtures and various other concoctions for at least a year.

To illustrate what dispensing was like in those days and what running a rural practice was really like, I should relate my experiences in two or three locums which I did in the interval between my father's illness and the locum with the Bradleys.

I arrived in Galway, on the west coast of Ireland, in a small town in a farming area. The doctor, an older man, was ready to leave when I arrived. He showed me the pharmacy, gave me a few quick tips and then gave me the keys of the car and said, 'Always have them bring in a urine specimen.' He added, 'Don't let anyone in here without a urine specimen'. I said, 'What tests do you want me to do on it?' He replied, 'It's not the tests I want it's the bottles, for the medicine.'

Doing another locum I learned one very important lesson and that was never to make up medicine in a screw-cap bottle. I had a patient come in with stomach trouble and a bad cough. I made up cough mixture and because of his acid stomach I added bicarbonate of soda, shook the bottle, screwed on the cap and gave it to him. He thanked me, put the bottle in his hip pocket and cycled away. In 20 minutes he was back. The bottle had exploded in his hip pocket and now I had to dress his backside. From then on corks were the order of the day.

My courtship of Gloria Bradley, the daughter of the elder Dr Bradley, continued and I made frequent visits to the Bradley home. Old Mrs Bradley was very interested in the progress of the practice and also very interested in marrying off all her daughters, and she was especially anxious that I should marry Gloria. When I told her that the practice was not really flourishing and that I was not really making much money, or getting my overdraft at the bank cleared, she told me that her husband would want me to join up with her son in the practice when he retired. She said that although my practice was not doing well I would do very well when I joined the Bradleys.

It was years later that I discovered that she and Dr Frank Bradley had not spoken to each other in a generation and that she had caused him much grief, to the extent that their two eldest children had been brought up by their grandparents. Old Mrs Bradley was an alcoholic and a drug addict. What she was telling me about what her husband had told her was nonsense and a figment of her imagination.

Gortin was at its best on a fair day, once a month, when the main street was packed with cars, lorries, cattle, sheep, carts with pigs, calves, horses, foals and some vegetables all for sale. Up and down the street there were lorries which opened up to display farm instruments, tools, chain barbed wire, etc., anything which could be useful on a farm. The fast talkers kept changing the prices on bargains. They would open a box of tools and bring their price down to get their sale started and when they had got to their lowest price they would say, 'That's it' and sell them for ten minutes. Then they would open another box and begin again with something different.

There were three-card trick men playing the shell game and 'trick-o-loop', all out to make a quick shilling or half-crown at the expense of what they thought were gullible farmers. Towards evening the crowd thinned out and ended up in the pubs, which was probably the only good day's business the pubs did in a month.

On a non-fair day you would come into Gortin and see nothing. It looked like a ghost town, maybe with one or two people walking or talking outside one of the four or five grocery stores but rarely outside a pub. There were about five pubs in town and other than on the fair day you would find nobody inside, not even the bartender, but if you hit the bell on the counter someone would come.

If anyone went into a pub for a drink they could easily be found because someone from across the street, although invisible, would see whoever entered or left. With hopeful anonymity one could drive one's car through the entry beside the pub into the backyard and park there, entering through the back door. All pubs had yards in the back where on a fair day cattle, carts and cars could be parked for a nominal sum. If one stayed too long in a pub one was considered to be drinking too much.

Before getting my house I entered and left the home where I stayed by the back door with my car parked in the backyard. It was easy then to slip in the back door adjoining the house where I lived and the pub owned by my landlady's mother and her husband. When I came home late and dinner was over in Johnny's house, I could go over to Mrs Loughran's pub and she would put up a fried meal with strong tea or bottle of stout in next to no time. She was from Donnegal and she spoke Irish. I spoke Irish too, so we had a very close almost mother to son relationship. Jimmy, her husband, was a dour Derryman but kindhearted and full of tales of the old days when he was young and ran barefoot in the Sperrins.

On the road going east to Carrickmore there was a very respectable pub which was well kept and to which a grocery store was attached. The owner was Paddy McCullogh of Greencastle. He was a politician and a businessman and kept an extremely clean and proper house. East of Greencastle there were no more pubs until one arrived in Carrickmore.

Going north from Greencastle, which was at the crossroads, there was a pub in a place called Glen Hull, a glen surrounded by mountains. The pub was manned only when a customer arrived. The owner was a pleasant old man and as he was a patient of mine I rarely passed without checking him out. His Guinness was not of the best because his turnover was sometimes slow.

On the weekends I occasionally would run into one of his regular customers called Mickey Gillen. Mickey had a peg-leg. He reminded me of Long John Silver in *Treasure Island*. He was more adept on that peg-leg running through a bog or over a mountain than I was with two legs. I am sorry that I did not record some of his stories of the years gone by because they were very funny and he was very droll. I often had to bring him to his mountain home when he was not in a fit condition to walk. As his amputation was above his knee he had to take his leg off to get into the car and then put it on again before he could get out. He was illiterate but he could count his money and multiply and divide quicker than anyone I ever knew. He also knew everything about everybody: who their ancestors were, who they married, who their doctor was, where they bought their groceries and where they went to church.

Mickey's cottage was out in the middle of a bog but accessible by car as long as the weather was dry. Whenever I had time to spare I would visit him when I was in the area and take him a six-pack of Stout and have one with him. I decided to get him a new leg one time and sent him to Belfast to get fitted. They gave him about two legs with a bending knee and all the latest contraptions but he always ended up with his peg-leg with which he was more comfortable. The prosthetists (leg makers) in Belfast finally agreed that he did better on the peg-leg so they made him a new one and for this he was extremely grateful. It was very comfortable and much lighter than his old one.

Halfway between Gortin and Omagh there was the Halfway House, which was very clean and a well-run pub which also served meals. It was whitewashed annually and there was plenty of parking in front. It was probably the closest thing to an English pub in that area. The bar, like Paddy McCullogh's, was well appointed with a comprehensive selection of spirits as well as beer and wine.

Once one crossed the Gortin Gap there was an almost puritanical disapproval, in that area, of drinking or of anyone who frequented the pubs or spent any length of time in one. However, there was a fairly brisk industry related to the making of poteen, or moonshine. One story told of an underground mine in Glenlark. The road came to a dead end in the glen, about where the mine had been. There was a still in the bottom of the mine but the police never seemed to be able to find the mine or the mouth to it. It was apparently well camouflaged by a slab or it might even have been under a house. I never got to see it but I was told the story.

In the days before cars the police travelled in horse-drawn sidecars, or traps, and one time they made an unexpected raid on a distiller up in the Glenlark area. They searched the house and the surrounding barns and stables and byres (the latter is a cow's house) but no poteen was to be found, although they could smell it. Before leaving they watered their horse at a raintub or an overflow barrel at the end of the house and left. About 100 yards down the lane from the house the horse staggered and fell. It could not be aroused and the smell of poteen on its breath was an immediate clue to where the poteen had been hidden. By the time the police got back to the house the tub was empty and the evidence gone. The farmer offered the police the use of his horse to get them back to town and looked after their horse until it sobered up. It is said that the farmer's wife killed a chicken and gave the police a meal and that they had a drink of whiskey for the road.

Another story told was that there was a large sewer behind the police barracks in Gortin and when a haul was made of poteen, the Superintendent of Police came out from Omagh and ceremoniously poured the poteen down the sewer. What he did not know was that a milk churn had been placed beneath the grating which would catch enough poteen to be served at a celebration in the barracks after the Superintendent had departed.

* * *

Dr Quinlivan in Carrickmore was a great friend. When he went away and I covered his practice for him he paid me generously but he would not hear of me paying him when he covered my practice. I visited him frequently as he was great company and fun to be with. Carrickmore, the town in which he lived and practised, had at least five pubs. If Dr Kevin was not at home he was in one of them and he was usually in the one outside which his Land Rover was parked.

On fair days in town, Kevin ran his practice from an upstairs office, the steps to which were outside the building. In good weather the waiting room was the steps outside. Kevin carried a prescription pad in his pocket and when he was stopped in the middle of the street he renewed his prescriptions there and then. I even saw him laying the prescription book on the back of a cow – which was tied to a lamp-post – while he was writing on it. He was famous throughout the area for being an excellent physician.

He was very kind and had a capacity for whiskey second to none. His medical acumen never seemed to suffer and he was always available night or day and his patients loved him. If he was sitting in a pub when a patient wanted to see him, the pub would always clear the back room, which then became Kevin's consulting room. When visiting him I once helped him examine a patient lying on a table in the back room of a pub.

When he first bought the Land Rover, because he was the doctor, he had been given a council house in a new estate outside town. Off the main road to the left there was a hill up to his house. One night coming in late, Kevin turned his new Land Rover left up the hill but he had not closed the car door properly and he fell out. The Land Rover continued up the hill and ended up against the front gate of his home. His wife, hearing the car arriving and seeing the lights but no sign of Kevin, went to find the car had come home without him. This was reminiscent of the old stories of the horse making its own way home without the horseman. When Kevin eventually walked up the hill and saw his wife standing there, he slapped the car on the bonnet and said, 'That's the kind of car I need. I'm glad I bought the old Rover.' He took the keys out of the car and went to bed.

Kevin's real hobby was greyhounds. He always had two or three which were trained by a trainer in a nearby town called Six Mile Cross. Whenever they thought a dog was well trained and ready to race, he would hire a limo and the carload would head for the Belfast racetrack.

He was quite wealthy and had no respect for money but he did enjoy backing dogs with the bookies and he had a strong lust for gambling. I was covering his practice when he went on these trips so I rarely went with him. One Friday afternoon he called me to tell me that he was on to a real sure thing and that he was taking the limo to Belfast and wanted to bring as many trustworthy people with him as he could to lay off the bets with the bookies. All the bets had to be laid on simultaneously because if a lot of money went on one dog the odds would immediately drop. He got a friend of his from Omagh to cover both practices because it was summer and business was slack.

We arrived in Belfast just in time for the race in which his dog was entered, even though we had stopped in several pubs along the way. Kevin doled out the money, giving each of us a £5 note. This was a lot of money in those days. He might have given some of the others £10 because they were experienced punters. Each one of us was to get in front of a bookie at the last moment before the race and slap on the money. I was placed in front of one bookie's stand and the others scattered right along. There must have been 20 bookies at that meeting. The dog's odds increased as nobody was backing it and it went up to 12 to 1, then 14 to 1, and when it got to 20 to 1 as a complete outsider Kevin gave the word 'Slap it on.' Immediately the odds came down to even money, the bookies suspecting that this was a sure winner. Winner it was. It was so far ahead of all the field that there could have been no question of a protest or any way to get out of it. Each of the backers got at least £100 back. This was in the middle of the meeting but Kevin wanted no more of that. We collected the dog, got into the car, out of the parking lot and headed for home before the pubs would be closed.

The last pub we visited was in a town called Dungannon and everyone was hilariously high by the time we left. Some in the party knew of a late house that we could get in after hours (closing time then being 10.30). When we arrived in the 'sheebeen' we were out of luck. There were no spirits but the publican had some Guinness stout. An older man with us had a peculiar taste for ether and had some. At one time it was legally bought over the counter in hardware stores and in worse and poorer days it was the only drink available for some of the poorer classes. However, the law had changed and it was discovered that it was an extremely dangerous drink. Some people went home, had a drink of ether and belched in front of the turf fire, causing an explosion that blew them wide open. Experienced alcoholics, however, could anticipate the danger signs.

The gentleman with us was experienced and knew when he was in trouble. After we had left the shebeen, he began to complain of severe bloating in his gut. The car was stopped and Kevin tried what would now be called the Heimlich manoeuvre, with no success. Kevin got the driver to drive on to the nearest house to get a rope. A horse's reins would usually be the easiest 'rope' to handle. We got to a house, banged on the door, and a man came to the window and asked what we wanted. Someone said we wanted a rope. The man said, 'Is it ether?' and they said 'Yes.' He rushed out to his stable, got a rope and we got the man with the bloating out of the car. They wrapped a rope around one leg and then gradually wrapped it around him tightly up to his chest. Kevin explained to me that the rationale of this was to keep the man from exploding. When he was thus protected from further expansion of his abdomen, they laid him on the ground and rolled him like a barrel. Suddenly the gas began to escape and the whole area smelled of ether. He belched and belched until I thought he would never stop. Finally, the rope got slack and the crisis was over. The farmer brought out some mashed potatoes and tea and told him to eat it. This brought up more gas and would prevent him from getting further problems.

When we got back to Carrickmore we got in the back door of one of the pubs and the celebrations continued until the small hours. My recollection of my lone drive back to Gortin is vague and fortunately there was very little traffic. New cars were rationed, as was petrol. I did not open my office on Saturday and that gave me time to get over my Belfast adventure.

Dr Kevin as usual was generous with his rewards to his co-conspirators. I have no recollection if the dog that won the money ever won another race. I cannot even recall its name but I am sure there are many bookies in Belfast who will never forget.

As I mentioned before, Gortin was a little town surrounded by mountains. The farming communities were scattered, and hard to reach, and because of the mountains, over which there were no roads, it was a long roundabout to reach some of the farms.

The government compensated a doctor by paying annual mileage depending on how distant the patient lived from the doctor's residence or surgery (as his office is called). The doctor was paid an annual fee, mileage and dispensing payment regardless of how many times he saw the patient. As the fee always remained the same, the patient never seen, or seen the least, was the most valuable. Ones seen often became less valuable with each visit. On the average, because of this the patients in distant areas could be worthwhile accepting on a doctor's panel. Some patients were worth more on mileage than on the basic fee.

I found that I spent more time on the road doing house calls than I did in my office, so I did my office hours early in the morning and the rest of the day doing house calls. There was no hospital nearer than 12 miles from Gortin and Derry city was 40 miles to the north. Everything from deliveries to heart attacks to pneumonias and everything non-surgical was treated at home. When someone needed an x-ray it would take 24 hours to get an ambulance to pick them up and bring them home again – that is, if they were willing to get into an ambulance.

The ambulance in those days and in that area, as in most areas throughout Ireland, was at the time considered a sentence of death and an ambulance was almost synonymous with a hearse, except that people travelling in the ambulance were at least alive when going away. Many thought that if they were coming back in the ambulance alive that they were coming back to die. Patients who died in the hospital came back in the hearse, so a doctor who treated patients at home was a blessing even if his treatment was not successful.

There were few cars and fewer telephones and bicycles were the commonest form of transport apart from walking. People did walk long distances, especially on a fair day, sometimes 14 miles to a fair and 14 miles home again; maybe driving or walking cattle or sheep to be sold, and even transporting pigs in a horse and cart, leading the horse most of the way.

Some homes could not be reached by car and I would drive the car as near as possible and then take my medical bag and walk from half a mile to three miles into the mountains. This was best done by changing into Wellington boots, which I always carried in the boot (trunk) of my car. At night I would be met by someone bearing a lantern, usually kerosene, but electric torches were becoming available. The batteries in those days did not last long and sometimes failed before my return journey. In Ireland, however, the doctor was always fortified with a stiff glass of whiskey on arrival and before departure, with ample cups of tea always available. If one was hungry there was nowhere on earth where one could get a fry like an Irish bacon and egg and chicken with bread and butter, all home-made, although creameries were beginning to be popular. Irish creamery butter is now available anywhere in the world.

New patients who were not registered on my panel were still willing to pay, but I felt uncomfortable charging them high fees and I never sent bills. Were I hard-headed and charged more I could have done extremely well, which would have also applied to my subsequent border practice – which I will describe later.

The development of my periphery practice in the Plumbbridge and Sperrin area on the border of the Sperrin mountains encroached on another doctor, who did not take kindly to this, which all came to a head when he refused to give a death certificate for a patient who died suddenly in his area. In desperation the dead man's relatives asked me if I could help. I went and viewed the body, examined it thoroughly and could find no evidence of foul play. The patient was elderly and by the history had obviously died of either heart attack or stroke. He was lifting a heavy bag of potatoes at the time he dropped dead so I gave him a death certificate saying he had died of a myocardial infarction. This was the start of a war that would continue for the rest of my time in Gortin between me and the other doctor. He being Protestant and I being a Catholic made matters worse but it precipitated a flow of medical cards to my panel in the valley in which the death took place. Every relative of the dead man, near and far, joined my panel and these relatives canvassed other relatives, friends and neighbours. This gave my practice a considerable boost and spread my reputation as a 'good guy', undeserved but welcome.

My friendship with my landlord and his wife and children became stronger as time went by because eating breakfast, lunch and dinner, listening to the same radio programmes and being closely thrown together, it was bound to happen. His customers became my customers and he was of an old family in the district with many relatives all of whom came to him with their cars if they had them, and tractors which they all had, to be repaired. He was a droll, humorous man and people stopped in to talk to him. His mother-in-law owned the block in which his house was situated and she owned a pub over which she and her husband lived. People coming to the pub who had horses or cattle stored them in the yard behind the pub and cars and tractors were also left there until Johnny could get to repair them.

During World War II Johnny had worked in Derry city with the 'Yanks', as the American troops were described. He was a superb mechanic and mechanical diagnostician. He was not on the make, never rushed a job and never sent a car out but that he would guarantee his repairs. I had access to his garage after he taught me how to do repairs. After I got rid of the Sunbeam Talbot in London and got my new Morris Minor, I continued to do valve-grinding jobs, greasing jobs, lubrication and all the maintenance on the Morris Minor that needed to be done. He showed me how to undertake modifications in the engine so that I won a hill climb in my class in the annual Fintona Hill Climb two years in succession. I was never sure if it was our modification or the addition of ether to the petrol just prior to the attempt on the hill. Johnny gave me a grounding on the basics of car maintenance, carburetter adjustment etc. that has lasted me until today, if I had the facilities and the inclination to undertake them.

When I met him Johnny was over his wild days in Derry with the Yanks and had some wonderful stories to tell of his friends among the Americans and of the strange things they did. Since coming to America and getting to know American ways, I now realize that many things that were strange to Johnny are not strange at all to me any more.

For instance, he could not understand eating bacon and eggs and having pancakes with syrup on the same plate. He had been a hard drinker in his day but he could not understand drinking down a straight whiskey or bourbon then following it with a beer. He loved the American mechanical ability. It was with the Americans that he first saw ratchet wrenches, ring spanners and power tools. Probably his adoption of all these methods contributed to his success and his speed in doing his work. When I met him, Johnny had dried out completely although he smoked heavily, as we all did. The fact that he was 'dry' was a blessing when some of the young businessmen and I occasionally went away for an evening on a motoring trip across the border into what they called the 'Free State'. This was the Republic. The pubs stayed open there until 10.30 p.m., and if one was a traveller from more than three miles distant one could drink until midnight without it being considered after hours.

On these trips Johnny was the driver. The local chemist, who came to the town after I had set up my practice, was one of our passengers, including two grocers and another publican. Johnny knew all the roads and back roads to the various fun joints, one of which included Pettigoe in the Free State. This is the nearest to St Patrick's purgatory, otherwise known as Lochderg, where penitents go during the spring or summer to spend three days starving, praying and walking around in their bare feet. Drunks go there sometimes to dry out because when you are on the island there is no way you can get out until you have done your 'penance'. Pettigoe has many shops selling holy souvenirs, rosaries, medals, scapulars and all the Catholic paraphernalia avidly bought by the sinners who have recovered and done their penance.

There is a pub for every holy shop, however, so when we travelled to Pettigoe with Johnny we visited them all. One of them is situated on the border, and half the pub is in the Free State and half of it is in Northern Ireland. There is a white line in the middle of the bar and prices are different if you are on the northern side or the southern side. At the time we were travelling, drinks were cheaper in the south so we sat on the south side of the line.

Frankie McConnel was the son of a local grocer. He was in pharmacy school when I set up my practice in Gortin and when he finished he opened a pharmacy in the town. I could have continued to dispense in spite of his presence but he was a very nice young man and to give him a start in the town which he loved, and in which his family lived, I discontinued dispensing – but not in time, unfortunately, to offset the impending disaster which would change my whole life.

Jackie, his brother, was working with his father in one of the biggest grocery stores in the area. Brian and Kevin McGarvey, who had another grocery store in the town, completed the party who travelled with Johnny across the border. These were hilarious trips but it was all good clean fun. The comfort of travelling in Johnny's huge Austin 16 taxi was really a luxury and I was safe in that I could leave Dr Kevin covering my practice when I was away.

On one trip we observed a bottle of champagne in the pub in Pettigoe and someone mentioned black velvet. We decided to try it. This consists of a bottle of stout with a shot of champagne added. There were only four of us, and four shots of champagne seemed like very little, so we divided the champagne four ways with four bottles of stout. It certainly tasted like velvet but we had had some drinks before this, not having passed by a pub without stopping. Well, things went from bad to worse and that was the end of the night. Johnny said it was the quietest night he had ever had – until he got back and tried to get us out of the car. We were all asleep and in no condition to go home, except for me. I was then renting the apartment and only had to go upstairs. Everyone else slept in Johnny's sitting room until daylight.

I had been a member of the Omagh Motor Club from early on in my time in Gortin because my first car, which I described earlier, was supposedly a sports car, but it was really a glorified Hillman with a Sunbeam Talbot body which I had bought second-hand in Belfast.

When I got my new Morris Minor I began to take part in motor crosses and trials seriously. It was grossly underpowered but it was new and drove well and was fairly manoeuvrable. The big event of the year was the Sion Finn Hill Climb, which was run in the hills between Fintona and Five Mile Town. The hill climb would be run in early summer and spectators would picnic along both sides of the road. There being no hedges, they could see the road from the fields.

The first year I entered, my car was new and I won my category. Johnny had tuned up the engine and we figured by adding a bottle of ether we could pep it up further. There was only one grade of petrol in those days, which was low octane, probably in the mid to upper eighties. As there were no new cars in my category it was an easy win.

The members and the competitors were a jolly bunch of men. Some of them were dentists, doctors, garage proprietors, mechanics, and one year it was attended by a newspaper executive from Belfast. His name was Bobby Baird and he was famous in the British Isles for his interest and participation in hill climbs and races of all descriptions. His anecdotes and opinions kept us all fascinated for most of the day.

The dinner which was held after the meet was always an hilarious affair. It was in Omagh, usually in the Royal Arms Hotel. The bar remained open after hours, the police turning a blind eye because many of them partook in the hill climb and the hilarity.

My brother Kevin, a doctor from Waterford, never missed the meeting and was extremely popular. His first entry was a Volkswagen into which he had transferred a Porsche engine. It performed way beyond anything else in its class and it was the only Volkswagen in Northern Ireland at that time. They had just started coming in from Germany to the Republic, but being such a revolutionary design had not yet begun to sell well. The engine at the back and being air-cooled, and the car having a heater, placed it completely beyond the imagination of people in the Republic. They were used to English Fords, Morrises and Austins. The

Morris Minor was as yet still a very big change from what had been pre-war and post-war design in the British Isles.

Another year, Kevin arrived with a Delage into which he had put a Hudson engine. On a straight road 100 miles an hour was well within its capacity. It had been fitted with a bypass for the exhaust system and when one got away from the city and the bypass switch being pulled, it sounded like an aeroplane because the muffler was non-existent and flames jumped out from the side of the car. It looked as though it were on fire. It was not well-tuned so it did not have any real success in hill climbing, but it certainly elicited an awful lot of interest.

The day after the hill climb, Kevin and I and his wife headed back to Waterford, where we had decided to take a vacation. We passed through Dublin and spent a while there and then set out for Waterford on a Sunday evening.

We decided we would let the racing car go first, with the other two cars – his wife driving the Volkswagen and my Morris Minor – following in the rear in case anything went wrong. Nobody would know if the racing car was behind us and it broke down. We took turns driving it because it was getting cold and there was nothing but the windscreen to protect the driver. Outside Naas, County Kildare, the inevitable happened. We ran out of petrol. The tank on the Delage was no match for its appetite for petrol. We were about one mile outside Naas in the middle of horse-racing country. We headed into Naas to see if we could buy petrol but no garage would open for us. This was about 1.30 or 2.00 in the morning. There was nothing for it but to siphon, and we had petrol cans.

Outside a hotel there were a lot of cars parked, so we picked one which was in the middle where we would not be seen. We got a tube, which we never went anywhere without, and got the siphon moving. We then went away and left the siphon running and came back when we thought the can was nearly full. It was overflowing when we returned but we had two gallons to bring back to the Delage, which we started and drove back into town. After several more siphoning sorties we had enough, we thought, to get us to Waterford.

There must have been some surprised guests the following

morning going out to find their tanks depleted. We hoped that their petrol indicators were accurate or there would be many people stuck on the highways.

We attended several other climbs but the car never won anything worth mentioning. My young brother was visiting Kevin once and Kevin brought him out to try and teach him to drive. While zooming down the road, a wide lonely road with no traffic, the young man changed into first gear instead of fourth, leaving bits and scraps of gearbox behind him. I think that was the demise of the Delage with the Hudson engine.

My next unusual car was a Renault, for which I traded the Morris Minor. Renaults were also an innovation, rear-engined with great acceleration and many advances in design and suspension. Shortly after I obtained it I left Gortin and moved to Fermanagh and did not get a chance to try it in a Fintona Hill Climb. The fate of this Renault will come later.

2

Married Bliss and Addiction

My practice continued to increase gradually but there was one snag. Patients who joined my panel after 1 April were not included on my list until the beginning of the next quarter, which would have been July. After 1 July I was not paid for new patients until after 1 September. I looked after some patients to keep them on my panel even though their previous doctor was getting paid for them. However, I felt I could support a wife by the middle of the summer of 1951 so Gloria and I got married in September of that year.

The marriage was in Dublin and we spent some of our honeymoon in Jersey in the Channel Islands, and the rest in Ireland. The house, though small, was adequate for both of us and in September 1952 our son Garvan was born. He was premature but he thrived remarkably well, partly because we gave him the wrong formula, which was too strong. He should not have started that formula until he was over 7 pounds. When we discovered the mistake we continued it anyway and he was one jump ahead of expectations from then on.

Shortly after we were married, Gloria developed a gluteal abscess on her right side. I did not know what it was until one day it began to show as a boil and then as a deep sinus. I gave her injections of penicillin, which cleared it up, but some weeks later she developed another one near the same area. I brought her to a doctor in Omagh, but he could not explain how this happened. She then developed a urinary infection, which entailed her going to the Royal Victoria Hospital in Belfast for a week of complete investigation and treatment.

I tried to visit her there twice a week, making the trip to and from Belfast, about 80 miles each way through all kinds of weather. On my way back from one visit I ran into a flood when I was doing about 60 miles an hour and my Morris Minor planed on the surface, turned around and rolled over. It took two months to repair and was never the same again. After that it was my first experience with motorcycles, and I became quite an expert at travelling the bad lanes, some of which I could not negotiate with a car anyway, but most places I could bring the motorbike to the door, so it had its advantages.

Gloria then developed what I thought was morning sickness and was vomiting so much one evening that I had to bring her to the hospital and leave her overnight. I got very angry when I heard some of the nurses whispering behind a curtain in the ward that she was drunk. With later developments, I came to realize that they were not far off the mark. She kept getting sick and got another abscess, although all pregnancy tests were negative.

One cold wintery February day shortly after we suspected that Gloria was pregnant, I got a call to a little hamlet called Roosky, about 4 miles out of town, to see Joe O'Neil urgently as he had a severe pain in his chest. When I examined Joe it was obvious that this man in his seventies had had a heart attack. I opened my bag to get some morphine and atropine, which came in rubber-stoppered bottles and which I always carried in my bag. All it needed was an injection of this to relieve his pain and perhaps carry him through the worst of the attack. There was no electricity in the house but there were Tilly paraffin lamps which his wife had brought to the bedroom. Taking out the rubber-stoppered bottle, I inserted a needle (I always carried a sterile syringe – they were reusable in those days) and found that the bottle was empty.

I searched frantically to see if I had another one, but there was no more. Fortunately I had a dissolvable morphine tablet for such an emergency. This was done by filling a teaspoonful with water, putting the tiny morphine atropine tablet in the water and holding it over a candle. When it came to the boil it was allowed to cool, taken into the syringe and injected.

This relieved Joe but he was going to need more injections through the night. I went home to get another fresh bottle of morphine atropine solution from my dispensary. I raced up the stairs and got out the box of morphine atropine bottles, which came in dozens. I had taken out about two. The first was empty. The next one was also empty, and the next. They had all been opened and the seal was not on any of them. To my horror I discovered that all the morphine was gone. I did not have any. It was late in the day and I would have to go to Omagh or somewhere where I could find a chemist open who would give me some more. I called George, who supplied me as a rule. His shop was closed and he had gone home.

I now had time to think about this situation and assess how it had come about. I asked Gloria if she knew how I had all these empty bottles. She denied all knowledge, saying she hadn't even known they were there. The only other explanation was that George had given me a used pack by mistake. I rang him at his home and he said that was impossible. He never gave me any packs that were not sealed. I remembered that this was true as they were always unopened when I got them. I remembered also that the bottle I had in my medical bag had been full when I took it out and I had used it several times over the previous months as there were ten injections in each bottle.

I tried to keep a cool head but I could feel this cold sweat and an empty feeling in my stomach and a strange feeling in the roots of my hair. It was dawning on me that Gloria had been using my morphine for I did not know how long and I had no idea in what quantities or how frequently.

I had really lived a protected existence all my life. I had lived as tho son of a doctor and for ten years I had lived in an environment of university pre-medical and post-medical in the presence of all types of diseases, students, house surgeons, house physicians and in a maternity hospital where drugs were used but always with great caution and with extreme economy.

During my university career a former medical student had described to the University Medical Society how he had become addicted to morphine while he was in a maternity hospital. He developed a toothache and a friendly nurse gave him a morphine tablet to put in the cavity to relieve the pain. Not having done anything about the tooth, after about six weeks he had left the hospital. However, he found himself going back to the friendly nurse in the hospital until the nurse became panicky, realizing what she had done. The young man had become a morphine addict. He was treated and sent to an institution in England, where he got the best of treatment and returned home cured. The paper on his problem which he read to the medical society was hailed as a wonderful presentation of the description of morphine addiction. He got the gold medal that year during the inaugural for his presentation. He continued his medical career but in two years he was dead from an overdose.

There were various rumours of doctors on staffs of various hospitals, especially anaesthetists and otolaryngologists, who were supposed to be addicted but no proof of it ever came out. There were alcoholics who showed themselves up at the annual medical society dance in the Gresham Hotel or at other similar functions, but even they were few and far between.

All this had cemented in my conscious and subconscious mind a horror of addiction, no matter to whom it occurred, but the horror was multiplied a thousandfold by realizing just the possibility that my beloved wife, whom I had married a few months ago, was an addict. Now I remembered the abscesses and the vomiting and the remarks in the hospital by the nurses, who could look at her objectively and not with a bias like I did.

After a long denial Gloria finally admitted that she had taken the injections once or twice but I could only reason that she had taken everything that was available, including some that was in my medical bag.

I could think of nothing else. I couldn't think of patients, I couldn't think of problems, all I could do was to get her into the car and drive her to Fintona and confront her father with the situation. He didn't seem surprised or horrified, which surprised and horrified me. Her brother came in and I told him the situation and he said, 'Well, you married her and she's your problem now, don't be annoying Daddy.'

I never did find out if they thought or knew that she was addicted even before I married her, but looking back I now realize that they were acquainted with the situation with her mother and this was their skeleton in the closet. It was as if they were waiting to see how soon I would discover what was going on and it was significant that the old lady, Gloria's mother, was never at any stage brought into the conference, such as it was. 'Such as it was' stems from the fact that it all took place in the small dining room in the Bradley home, everyone standing up, with old Dr Bradley looking out of the window with his back to the fire. Neither he nor Dr Seamus addressed each other. The old man was a man of few words anyway and this evening he had fewer than ever. As far as I can recall, neither of them spoke to Gloria to admonish her or to ask her if this was true.

Looking back, I realize that what I should have done was to have taken Gloria and gone to my parents in Dublin. My father would have given me a sympathetic hearing and would certainly have taken it upon himself to do something, although he probably would have known then, as I know now, that Gloria was already a lost cause. My father, however, was a highly qualified doctor who had earned the highest degree possible in medicine in the British Isles, the MD. He was a former President of the Medical Society in University College, Dublin, and a member of the Irish Academy of Medicine, and right in the middle of active up-to-date medicine both in Dublin and London. Later he would become President of the Irish Medical Association.

I had turned to what I can now see was a pair of country buckwheat doctors who had never upgraded their medical knowledge and whose main interest was to get me to hell out of their house, out of their lives and out of their way. Never again, as long as I was in Ireland, did they mention the subject or ask me how I was dealing with it or how they could help.

Some three years later, when I was in my second practice, Dr Bradley senior called me and asked me to come to see him. I had no idea what he wanted but I had hoped that some day he might invite me to join the practice and this might be the time.

He had built a new house across the street from the original. It was a small bungalow in which he, his wife and Marie lived. The reason he had left the big house was to have it available for Seamus when he, Frank, retired Seamus could then take over with the minimum of hassle and bring in a bride if he married.

When I arrived he looked grave and extremely worried. He told me that when his salary cheque arrived that morning it was much reduced. He had called Belfast to find out why and they told him that Dr Seamus, his son, had changed the percentage of the practice. Seamus had sent all the signed medical cards showing that now two-thirds were in his name and one-third in his father's name. His father, of course, was not aware that Seamus had been having them changed all along. The relationship was reversed and the son was now the owner of the practice and the father the junior partner.

There was little I could do but I understood that I was the only one that Frank could speak to about it and he had to speak to someone. Most of his previous friends and associates had died or left the area and retired. I tried to console him and I suggested that he retire. That was the worst blow, because if he had retired prior to this changeover he would have had three times the pension which he would now get. Seamus had foiled that as well as reducing his salary if he had stayed on.

I was not surprised, however, because I knew that Seamus had been changing cards. He had apparently waited until he had sufficient to send them all to Belfast and do the whole thing in one go. I had been getting to know Seamus over the years and found him to be selfish and uncaring but an extremely good businessman.

I went to see him and told him what his father felt about the situation and how shameful I thought his action was. He told me to go to hell as it was none of my business and if I thought that I would ever get into the practice I had another thought coming. He said that he knew that I was angling around to try to get in but as long as he now had control of the practice that would never happen. It all bore out my feeling that he was cold and calculating. I had never heard him speak warmly of his family. He despised his parents and his sisters. He was openly critical of almost anything they did.

When he married, he married the daughter of a rich businessman in Belfast and it was obvious that she was 100 per cent behind him when he stole his father's practice.

Dr Frank did not live long after that, dying suddenly within two years.

* * *

The Fintona Golf Club was a very active club and had all the gentry of the town as members. I had been a member while I was doing the locum and I remained a member all through the years. The Captain's Night was always great fun, when the Captain's Prize for golf was presented. The ladies made buffet-type edibles and there was lots of whiskey and beer etc.

In the year after Seamus switched the practice, Gloria and I and Dr Kevin Curran and his wife attended the Captain's Night party. When we entered the club, Dr Seamus shouted across the room that they didn't want interlopers like me and Dr Curran coming from the outside to drink the free booze. As it happened, Dr Curran and I had brought enough for ourselves and our wives to drink, and more. I shouted back at him, 'Are you going to steal the golf club like you stole your father's practice?' He attacked me but got nothing out of that but a black eye, which I gave him. There was chaos in the club and Seamus left shouting, 'I'm going to tell Daddy what you did and said.' I never heard what Daddy said to him but the next time I saw his father he smiled and said, 'That was quite a black eye you gave Seamus.'

I never spoke to Seamus again and I never met him again. When we visited Fintona we visited his father and mother in Marie's house and we never again went back to Greenanne, the big house.

Whatever the town people knew about the machinations of the Bradley practice before, they now had the whole story and it was out in the open. People were asking questions and although I was not there to answer them, I am sure Marie and the old doctor got plenty of opportunity to explain what was the cause of the brawl.

My parents never heard about any of this until I was long out of Ireland and far beyond their help or the need of it, but they did assure me then, and I believe it was true, that they would have gone to the ends of the earth to help me. If that had happened this story might not be worth telling.

Much later, in 1962, Gloria appeared on Belfast Television and my parents saw her admitting to her addiction. That was when they realized why I had divorced her.

With the discovery of Gloria's addiction we had long talks

about the problem and she promised that this was the end of it and that she would never do it again. I was naive enough to believe that this might be possible, but gradually it got through to me that it was not possible and there would be no recovery. She would get samples that came through the mail and try them even though they were not narcotics. She would try some of the medical ingredients in my pharmacy, which it was impossible to lock. I had to have a partition placed across the bathroom with a door and a lock. The carpenter, who was a patient and a friend, was obviously curious as to why I had him do that but I had to keep it a secret.

Morphine and pethidine which I needed to run the practice when on house calls I had to keep locked in my car. I had to bring my wife with me no matter where I went in the car as I could not leave her at home with all the medications in the pharmacy. She could still reach it. She would get up at night while I was sleeping, supposedly to go to the bathroom, and then had access to the tincture of extract of morphine. She would even take atropine and ready-made cough mixtures. I soon learned to notice immediately when she had taken anything as she developed an involuntary frown between her eyebrows and her personality and her conversation became different. I could not bring her in the car on maternity calls as sometimes I spent many hours waiting for a delivery. Even when the wooden partition was placed in the bathroom I always had to carry the key with me, and the occasional times that I did forget the key I came back to find that Gloria had been into the narcotics.

Life became a continuous running battle of accusations and denials because she never once admitted that she had taken medication of any description, even though it was quite obvious that she had. I decided to get the morphine and atropine in vials that had to be filed and broken to be used, and once I found a vial under her pillow, broken and used, but she denied that she had used it and said she didn't know how it got there. There was still nobody but us around with access to the drugs.

One evening I came home and found her unconscious in the bed and I was unable to waken her. Between the sheets I found a spilled half-empty bottle of powdered cocaine and a syringe. As I did not carry cocaine I had to ask Frank, one of the chemists I used, if he had any in stock and when he went to look for it it was gone. Yes, Gloria had been in his shop that day and he had gone into the back to look for something that she wanted and he had not noticed if she had gone behind the counter or not. His name was on the bottle so I had to tell him my predicament and advise him never to leave her alone in his shop again. The cat was out of the bag and I don't know how many people he told. I like to think that he kept the secret.

There was no possibility that I could ever get a house for rent or continue to live in the one I was in, so I had to decide reluctantly that I should have to move my practice and go somewhere else where housing was available and where I would not have to dispense in my home.

Every so often practices became available, usually from the death of older practitioners, in Northern Ireland. Doctors were notified of the vacancy in order that they might apply to fill it. Because the shop had now been shut, one could not move one's practice or set up in a different locality. Permission was needed from Belfast and outsiders could not come in to open up a practice.

When I notified the Ministry of my practice at the time that I applied to practise under the National Health Service, I filled in the form, and on the form there was a question 'Religion?' Being a Catholic and being young and having been brought up to believe that denial of one's religion was tantamount to going to hell after one died, I had written in 'Roman Catholic'. Being a Roman Catholic in Northern Ireland meant that one would not get one of the more lucrative practices, most of which were in cities and large towns. I was short-listed on many applications but of course was not granted any of them.

There was an elderly internal medicine specialist in Derry whom I had out on consultations, and on one such consultation I informed him of my predicament with Gloria and asked his advice. He said he was 70 years of age and had practised all over the world and that the only advice he could give me was to beat the hell out of her whenever I found her taking medication that was not prescribed. He was sorry for me, he said, and he would have advised immediate divorce but he knew that I was a Catholic and that I was locked in.

Divorce in those days was out of the question and I would not have considered it for myself or recommended it to anybody else. I could not have imagined that in seven years Gloria and I would be divorced. In spite of all her shortcomings, I still loved her and hoped that salvation would come from maybe a change of residence or some miracle, in spite of all the information and knowledge that I had that this was an incurable condition. I have always been an optimist and that was what carried me through and upheld me in the stormy years ahead. I was yet to learn of Gloria's mother's grim but closely kept secret.

In my youth and innocence there was another dreadful possibility which I had not entertained, in spite of finding Gloria comatose in our home from the stolen cocaine. A fatal dose of some narcotic was a very viable possibility, and looking back on it I cannot imagine why I did not take it into account. Had it happened I would be found guilty and possibly executed for her murder.

Trying to keep our problem a secret kept me from getting further advice because of trying to protect her from herself and from critics. Perhaps I carried some of the guilt myself for letting everything go so far and get out of hand because of my own carelessness. It was fortunate, or perhaps unfortunate, that when I bought narcotics I did not have to account for them or keep a log as I used them.

The enormous quantities of liquid narcotics which Dr Bradley senior had given me to open my pharmacy were unaccounted for anywhere, although he might have kept a log before the National Health Service started. When he closed his dispensary there was no system by which track could be kept of the medications.

Addiction in those days was a rarity. Drugs were not sold on the streets and problem addicts were registered with the Ministry of Health. They were supplied with drugs as needed so that an illicit market never developed.

Years later when I started work in Canada and in the United States, the tight surveillance and records kept in hospitals, nursing homes and elsewhere amazed me and brought me to realize that back in Britain and Ireland we were years behind in keeping records and controlling narcotics and preventing situations such as befell me.

3

Second Practice – Northern Ireland (1953–59)

The National Health system had only started in 1948 and had replaced the old panel system. As conditions improved, situations and salaries in England improved, but at that stage I had gone in a different direction.

The Chief Medical Officer from the Department of Health in Belfast visited all doctors annually and he visited me early in 1953. At this time the chemist had opened his shop and I had given up much of my dispensing practice, partly to give him a good start and partly to get my own dispensary out and get rid of the medications. This would eliminate the problem of having to watch Gloria and keep the dispensary locked and also the car. This reduced my income by one-third, as dispensing was profitable because the dispensing and mileage were paid whether a patient was seen or not.

I am not of a secretive nature, so when the Chief Medical Officer visited I thought that I would lay some guilt on him and I told him the whole story about Gloria's addiction, without telling him how far she had gone and how much medication had disappeared before I discovered the problem. It would have been leaving myself open to criticism and might have brought problems on myself for not keeping a closer eye on my supplies and having better records. I explained to him why it was vital that I get into a practice where I could get housing other than having surgery and office in my home. I think the Medical Officer was called Dr Robinson. He was very sympathetic and I told him that I had made many applications for positions for which I was short-listed but never appointed. He gave me a sidelong look which we both understood and said, 'Well, we both know why that was', implying that being a 'Papist' I hadn't a chance of getting to a more lucrative practice. He said, however, that he knew of a practice which was going to become vacant on the border in County Fermanagh, next to County Cavan in a town called Belcoo. He advised me to go and take a look and visit the doctor who was going to retire, a Dr Hamilton. He wanted me to keep in touch with him and let him know if I would be interested in the transfer, almost promising me that if I did apply I would get it.

On a fine day in May 1953 I had Dr Quinliven cover for me and I put Gloria and Garvan in the car. I drove to Fintona and left them there with her family and went on to see what it was like in Belcoo and Blacklion. Belcoo was on the north side of the border and Blacklion on the south side in the Republic of Ireland. I knew the country up to Enniskillen but from there to Belcoo I had never seen it.

Dr Robinson had told me that Dr Hamilton lived in Blacklion and that he had a dispensary on the southern side also. The practice in Northern Ireland was really not a very big one but that it was heavily subsidized by private practice in the south. The dispensary practice Dr Hamilton had occupied since before the Rebellion and the truce and establishment of the border between the north and south of Ireland. Petrol was very cheap in the Republic, so as soon as I crossed the border I immediately pulled up outside the first petrol pump, which was outside a pub. I had let the tank become as empty as possible before I arrived. I went into the pub to get someone to fill my tank, and that was my first meeting with Philip Dolan and the beginning of a long friendship and some hilarious encounters with the town 'character'.

To break the ice I ordered a pint of Guinness from this completely bald-headed man with a red face, aged about 53 and standing behind the bar with his arms folded. He pumped a pint and he knew I was a stranger, of course. It was a fair day and the town was full of people and cattle. Cars on both sides of the street were nose in to the pavement and there was hardly room to get in or out. I told him I wanted some petrol. He folded his arms and stood behind the bar and looked at me and said, 'Well, that's that.' He rolled his tongue around his lower lip and repeated, 'Well, that's that.' He said, 'Are you buying cattle today?'

I said, 'No, I'm a doctor.'

He raised his eyebrows and looked down his nose and said, 'Well, there's nobody sick in here, except the ones I make sick with that stuff.'

He threw back his head and laughed and then suddenly got a straight face, and I said, 'I hear that Doctor Hamilton is going to retire. Could you tell me where he lives?'

He took my pint off the top of the counter and put it through a little window on a shelf on the inside of the window in the 'snug' and said, 'You'd better sit in here.' So I went through a door and got into the snug and he stuck his head through the window and said, 'I'll have somebody to talk to you, and that's that.'

I said, 'I want to pay you for this.'

He said, 'Well, that's that.'

Next thing a young man with a big head of hair but well dressed came through the door and said, 'Philip tells me you're a doctor.'

'Yes,' I said, and introduced myself.

He said, 'I'm Mal O'Dolan, and don't pay any attention to Philip, he's drunk.'

I asked, 'Is Philip the man in the bar?'

'Yes,' he said. 'He's Philip Dolan,' and he smiled and went on to say, 'This fair day is a big day for him, but he's never so drunk that he can't take the money.'

I told Mal that I was probably going to be applying for the position of doctor in the area. He told me he lived on the north side of the area and that the doctor from a dispensary 12 miles further into the Republic was covering the dispensary at the present time for Dr Hamilton.

Mal bought me another pint and finished his whiskey and I found him to be a very genuine upright young fellow who had inherited his father's farm. His father had died some years previously and he lived with his mother and the rest of the family. He suggested that I visit Dr Hamilton, who lived next door to Philip's pub. Having finished our drinks I said goodbye to Philip and Mal and paid for my round at least.

Dr Hamilton was a very pleasant gentleman and probably in his early seventies, grey-haired, with a nice face and ready smile. He introduced me to his wife who was probably in her sixties. He told me about the practice and about the neighbouring doctors, one in the north and one in the south. The one in the south was covering his practice in the north, a Dr Hawkins in a town called Dowra, which is on the border of Cavan and County Leitrum. The other, Dr McGuire, had a practice in a place called Florencecourt. Florencecourt was a mansion but it gave the name to the area around it. When I visited Dr McGuire, I found that his home and practice was out in the country with no village near it.

Dr Hamilton told me that it was a very pleasant place to live and he thought I would get all the patients on the north side of the border but he was not quite sure what would happen to the dispensary practice in the Republic, the side on which he lived. After thanking him for his information, I said goodbye, went back and filled my car with petrol. I had another pint with Philip and carried on a conversation with him which had neither head nor tail to it. I was later to find out that Philip spoke in a vernacular of his own, which over the years had been adopted by the village and the surrounding countryside.

When I was leaving the village, Mal flagged me down and advised me to call in at the Railway Bar up on the Belcoo side of the border. This was apparently where Dr Hawkins called, coming and going down to Belcoo when he was covering for Dr Hamilton.

I stopped in at the Railway Bar and met Mae McGovern, and told her what I was doing. She was very interested and very helpful and introduced me to lots of people in the pub. It was busy because of the fair day on the Blacklion side. She put up a hearty meal and, like Philip, she would not take any payment. She was very encouraging and thought that I could make a good living and said she would do anything she could, even so far as to get housing for me.

It was nightfall when I left Belcoo. When I arrived in Fintona to pick up my wife and son, I spoke to Dr Bradley Senior and told him what I had in mind and why. I told him of my talk with Dr Robinson, and he considered it a good idea because he knew Dr McGuire and Dr Hamilton well from the old days. He said he would telephone them and find out what the situation was from their angle.

The next weekend I went to visit Dr Bradley Senior again, and he said that everyone recommended strongly that I move. They would give me every assistance and help me to get established in the area.

I promptly applied for the position and the Ministry confirmed my appointment. I was told how to resign from Gortin and what to do with the records of my patients (send them to Belfast), so I promptly started to get ready to move.

It was difficult and embarrassing and guilt-producing telling my patients that I was leaving. Really leaving them in the lurch, because those of them who had changed their cards to get on my panel would possibly have to try and get Dr Clark to take them back, or get doctors from other areas to look after them.

I was the bad boy in Gortin from then on and even my friends were cool. The only one who understood my predicament was Frank the chemist, and I told him that he could blow the gaff when I was gone and explain about my private problems and Gloria's addiction.

Small cars were absolutely unobtainable in Northern Ireland, although large cars like a Lee Francis, which Seamus Bradley had bought, and Armstrong Siddleys, which my former girlfriend's husband had and big cars like Austin A90s, which were very expensive, could be bought. These were being purchased by doctors better off than I.

I could not afford such a big car, however, but I happened to see an advertisement in Derry city for Renaults which were to be imported from France. Having given up my practice, I had time to go to Derry and investigate. They could get me a Renault 750, a rear-engine car, in two weeks, and while I was there I had a drive in one. To get them on the road they were giving an unbelievable offer for my Morris Minor so I arranged the exchange.

It was fun driving back and forth from Gortin to Belcoo in the new car. A retired schoolteacher in Belcoo was collecting medical cards for me in the medical office which he had been renting to Dr

Hamilton. I took over the rental, spent some time there and saw some patients. Before the end of June I had collected some 700 to 800 medical cards. I made the mistake of not taking them all and bringing them to Belfast and registering them in my name before 1 July. Not having them registered with the Ministry, I could not begin to get paid on them until 1 September. However, I was paid in July for the medical cards which had been in my name in Gortin for the previous quarter.

There was no housing available in Belcoo at all so I got established in the local hotel, which was run by an elderly lady and her daughter. The food was excellent and I had a lovely room with two windows looking out on the lake. Belcoo is situated between two lakes which are between Northern Ireland and Eire. Upper Lake MacNean drains into the Lower Lake MacNean through a small short river on which there was a weir for fish to pass up prior to spawning.

Belcoo is an L-shaped town north of the border. The short arm of the L is the beginning of the road to a border town called Garrison. The long arm is the beginning of a road that goes on to Beleek, another border town, where the Beleek china factory operates.

Beleek is on the border between County Fermanagh and County Donnegal, the latter being in the Republic and about 8 miles from Bundoran, a large seaside resort with a championship golf course and many first-class hotels.

Garrison, which is about 20 miles from Belcoo, is also a stopping-off place for fishermen who fish Loch Melvin and is world-famous for salmon fishing. Belcoo is a centre for fishing, golfing and touring the north-west of Ireland. It is mountainous but not as ruggedly mountainous as Gortin. I was to find out that very few of the homes were not within reach by car.

My 750 Renault had a good underneath clearance and lived up to its descriptions in the car magazines as climbing like a cat. Being one of the first Renaults in Ireland it was also a source of great interest and admiration. Its colour, a metallic beige, was also an original.

The practice got off to a good start. Dr Hamilton had the community well trained in that he had surgery hours between 11.00

a.m. and noon in Belcoo every morning, none at weekends and no afternoons or evenings. Dr Hamilton's practice was being looked after by a Dr Hawkins from Dowra and he had been doing the surgery in Belcoo. He also covered the surgeries in Dowra, Blacklion and Glenlevin. He anticipated applying for Dr Hamilton's dispensary practice. A dispensary practice is a salaried position, run by the Republic of Ireland, supplying medication and medical attention free for the indigent.

There were few, if any, indigent in the area, however, as many of them were wealthy farmers running small farms. Many of them had been to the United States. After spending some years there they had come home again with money, and many had relatives in the United States who were sending home money.

The branch surgery in Glenlevin was in a very mountainous area which is famous for being the source of the Shannon River, the longest river in the British Isles. It has many lakes along it and wonderful salmon and trout fishing. Where the river originates in Glenlevin it is called the Shannon Pot and tourists like to go there and jump across, saying they jumped across the Shannon, which in certain places might be the widest river in the British Isles. The town was then blessed by at least four pubs, one of which was next door to the post office and the others were in houses in the hills. There was a police barracks, a church and a post office.

The police, known in the Republic of Ireland as civic guards, were very lenient as far as late hours in the pubs. There was only a sergeant and two civic guards in the barracks and they were not above visiting the pubs after hours themselves. There was a dance hall and the guards were busy on Sunday nights as the boys coming to the dance from the pubs frequently got into fights over girls, property rights, property lines, cattle trespassing and who knows what else.

The dispensary in Glenlevin opened two days a week and operated out of one of the pubs, called Johnny Mickey Ruadhs. The name meant that he was Johnny, the son of Mickey the red-haired McGovern. Almost everybody in Glenlevin was called McGovern.

I had left Gloria and Garvan in the Bradley home in Fintona and once a week I would make a trip to visit them. The Renault was proving very nippy on the bends between Belcoo and Fintona – a distance of about 30 miles over winding and mountainous roads. It was an hour's trip if no stops were made and no slow traffic encountered.

One Sunday I spoke to Gloria on the telephone and she told me that her brother Seamus was going to Bundoran for the day and she would go with him and bring Garvan, and I could meet them there. This I did and we had dinner and danced in the Great Northern Hotel in Bundoran. They had brought their sister Marie also and later they all went home.

I headed back also, having to go through Beleek because the border would have been closed along the short cut to Blacklion. A light rain had started and on a long, although fast, curve outside Bundoran, my nice new Renault got into a skid, turned around and rolled over. Something I had not known, but which I found out later, was that with Michelin X tyres, which were new on the market, they held marvellously and had great holding power until they came to their breaking point, when suddenly everything gave way and their holding power disappeared. This was at the time of the introduction of radial tyres, which had just come on the market, and they behaved completely differently than the old-fashioned tyres.

My car was completely wrecked. Not long after, while I surveyed the remains, a car came along and stopped. It was a band on their way back from a stand in Northern Ireland. Fortunately one of them had a garage in Bundoran. He went back for his towing equipment and towed my car back to Bundoran. He said he would start working on it the following morning. They drove me back to Blacklion because they could not get back across the border and I walked to the hotel across the bridge.

Being without transport, and rental cars not being available in that area in those days, I bought a motorcycle to get me around. It was a small motorcycle by today's standards, just 350 cc, but quite adequate. Being a two-stroke meant there was oil in the petrol, and I found that if I went for long distances using the windscreen, the engine would seize up, the back wheel would stop turning and it would throw me. After escaping death in two such episodes I realized what the cause was. The resistance of the windscreen had to be done away with and I would have to go without it. This gave me many cold and wet trips, but with plenty of rain gear I was able to continue.

I had another problem that I did not know about. The insurance company covering my car did not cover accidents in the Republic, and the small print in the policy indicated this too late. Had I known, I could have been covered by a small additional premium, but now it was too late. I was so overdrawn on my bank in Omagh that I dared not try to get any more money there.

One evening in Philip Dolan's pub I was telling him of my predicament and he volunteered to lend me the money to redeem the car when it was repaired. For this favour I became his friend and his petrol customer almost for the rest of my time in Blacklion. My car took two months to be repaired as parts had to be brought from England. There was no agency in the Republic of Ireland as yet because Volkswagen had claimed the market and nobody was interested in another similar car with no advantage over it. Volkswagen parts and service were available and cheap but nobody knew anything about Renaults.

About this time I was approached by a farmer, cattle dealer and sheep dealer who had built a house outside Belcoo for his son, whom he was hoping to marry off to a local girl. He said he would rent it to me as the son's girl had left for England and was not coming back. She was working in London and making a lot of money. It had been built by his sons, men of all trades, and certainly not masters of building. The doors didn't meet the floor and the whole building was of cement blocks with a corrugated iron roof that in places did not meet the walls. Even the front door had about an inch of space between it and the cement floor, which was not covered. There was no pathway to the road and the house was really in a field, which was fine in dry weather but when wet it was muddy. I had no choice, however, and the rent was reasonable, or rather I should say I could afford the rent. Actually, no rent would have been reasonable for this ramshackle. My furniture was still in Gortin, and as it was cheaper to pay the rent on the house than to pay storage, I wrote to my brother-in-law, who had a store near Fintona – and a lorry. He volunteered to bring help to move it into the new house.

John Henry was a great help and a very obliging young man. He would not take any money for the move. When he brought the furniture to Belcoo he said, 'You are mad to move into this and put good furniture in here. It won't last a year.' It was now too late; it was there, and there was some chance of Gloria and Garvan moving in with me. One thing was certain: there would be no drugs in this house.

There was no electricity, but the telephone company volunteered to put in a telephone. John Henry obliged as he had a country store and supplied me with good paraffin oil lamps. There was a stove, a black old-fashioned one, and it was a coal burner. There was nowhere to store coal except in a heap outside the door, and this did not add to the 'beauty' of the house. The truck that delivered the coal would not go around to the back of the house because they were afraid they would get stuck in the muck and then not be able to get out again. The house was part of the Scott farm complex and there were farm sheds around the house, and in one there were pigs which the Scotts were dry feeding. Too late I learned that the pigs went to eat whenever they were hungry. They could push a wooden slat and dry pig feed would come down and they would eat it. There were automatic water fountains which they could operate also and get something to drink. There were straw beds around for them to sleep on. All they did was eat, drink and sleep. Each day one of the Scott boys came and swept the cement floor out through the door and then hosed the floor out. The pig waste smelt strongly at first but after a while one got used to it and didn't notice it.

The oil lamps were a nuisance but we had one Aladdin lamp with a mantle which gave a very bright light. We found out the hard way that one must be very careful when using this kind of lamp and never leave it unattended. We came in one night, having been to a movie in Blacklion, to find the house looking very dim from the outside. When we got into the house everything was black. Soot covered everything we had. On things that were dark we could not see the soot but it was there. This was a breaking last straw as far as Gloria was concerned. She decided to go back to Fintona until we got better housing.

Having got some help, I got the place straightened out and I brought Gloria back to Fintona the next weekend. Most of our clothes had to go to the cleaners, even the bedclothes were ruined. I decided that I would at least continue to sleep in the house, but word of the disastrous conditions got around and one day I got a call from a Major Nixon to come to see him.

Major Nixon had a house on the Lower Loch McNean. It was called 'The Cottage' but really it was a big roomy house. It was one-storey and extended through the middle of a garden at the back and had a large gravelled driveway in front. While Major Nixon was sitting with his wife and having a whiskey after dinner, I visited. Of course he did not ask me to join them, but he asked me to sit down. He said that he had an apartment over the stables and garage in the back of his house. He had heard that my living conditions were pretty awful and that he and his wife had discussed it and felt I should look at it and see what I thought.

The flat was absolutely beautiful. There were two large rooms, one a sitting room and one a bedroom. The bathroom was very big, with electricity and running water, hot and cold, and there was a nice kitchen. There were fireplaces in both rooms, polished wooden floors and it had all been cleaned out and made extremely habitable. This was a heaven-sent reward, and of course I accepted it immediately, especially at the charge of one pound a week which was half of what I was paying Jimmy Scott for the pigsty.

John Henry again came to my rescue and moved me. By now we had our clothes and bedding back in acceptable condition and when I moved, Gloria came back. We were really falling in love with Belcoo, Fermanagh, the Nixons and starting a new lease of life. I had by now got my car back and my only worry was clearing my overdraft at the bank, which was now about £1,200 pounds, and paying off Philip, to whom I owed £500. The Ministry was now paying me on a quarterly basis and I was getting considerable private practice from south of the border.

Dr Hamilton had now left and Dr Hawkins had bought his house in Blacklion in anticipation of getting the dispensary. When the dispensary was advertised publicly for application I applied, hoping that I would get back on the same footing as Dr Hamilton:

half a practice in the north and half a practice in the south. However, because I was living in Northern Ireland, my application could not be accepted, and without checking further I presumed that if I moved and lived in the Republic I would lose my Northern Ireland practice, so I cancelled out and Dr Hawkins got the practice.

We remained on friendly terms and he even asked me to cover for him when he went on vacation, as I had asked him to do for me, knowing it was a one-way street. Nobody in Northern Ireland was going to pay Dr Hawkins when they knew they they could have free treatment from me, so although he could cover me while I was away, there was no likelihood that the patients would continue to stay with him. The opposite was not the case, however, because all the patients in the Republic were paying patients; nobody wanted to get the name of having free medical treatment, because this indicated that they were paupers.

This was the situation in most dispensaries in the Republic but the viability of the practice was maintained by keeping a turnover list of patients who were treated free. Although they were not treated free, their names were put on a list to submit to the government, justifying free medication and medical equipment. Dispensaries which did not have a proven need for their existence would be discontinued and closed down. There was also the possibility of the quantity of free medicines and supplies being curtailed. There was no law against giving a patient medication out of the free supply and charging. This was considered one of the perks and kept doctors practising in remote areas where the private practice could not make up for the poor salaries paid by the government. The bureaucracy that would be necessary to supervise an alternative would further increase the cost of running the dispensary system and render it less viable.

When I covered for Dr Hawkins while he was on vacation, many of the patients wanted to continue to have me as their physician, but this would have been unethical and poor medical etiquette. Patients got around this by having Dr Hawkins see them for two to three months and then changing over to me. It would have been unreasonable for me to continue to refuse to see them. Many of the homes to which I went in the Republic seemed to be in poor circumstances and I kept my fees to a minimum and frequently did not charge at all. This was a grave mistake. I should have remembered what Professor Meenan had said to the class before our last clinic and final examinations – 'If you charge your patients too little they will consider you cheap and will not thank you.'

Later, when I was leaving the practice in 1959, Jimmy McGovern told me, 'It was none of my business so I didn't say it sooner, but people said to me, McCann is cheap so he can't be any good.' He added, 'Dr Hawkins charged two to three times what you did and he sent bills.' I had never sent bills to my patients and that was my mistake. However, that's getting ahead of myself.

Gloria was pregnant again and in April 1954 Keevsa, our daughter, was born in the apartment at Major Nixon's. She was attended by Dr Smith of Enniskillen, otherwise known as TA, which I think stood for Thomas Anthony or something like that. TA was a taciturn old gentleman who was getting on in years and took life very easy. Never hurried or got excited. He was an excellent obstetrician, however, and there was never any likelihood of there being problems with the confinement.

The Northern Ireland practice flourished but it was limited by the population in the area, and I now discovered that expansion too far would be uneconomical even though I was again dispensing from Dr Hamilton's old dispensary. It was a lock-up and pretty safe from Gloria. One snag was that the waiting room was just a passage outside with no room for seating. People would sit in the cobbler's shop at the front of the building. There was always a fire in there and the cobbler liked the company. I eventually found a butcher's shop down in the main street which was only used once a week by a lady to bring fresh meat from Enniskillen. She had decided to close the operation and the owner gave me the first offer to rent it. I was able to separate it into a front and back with an adequate waiting room and a consulting room with a lock-up pharmacy built in. The owner volunteered to do all the alterations. I now had a very comfortable consulting room with a built-in desk and an examination table. In the old dispensary I was compelled to stand. I stood on one side of the desk and the patients stood on the other. In the event of having to examine them they would have to lie on the floor.

With the advent of the new surgery, life was more organized. I had a waiting room where patients could sit and wait if I was late. The lady who lived behind my new surgery had a key and would open the waiting room at 10.30 a.m., or earlier if there were patients, and I would start consultations at 11.00 a.m. and go until such time as everyone was seen. It rarely took over an hour. People didn't mind waiting as everyone knew everyone else and they could sit and gossip. Mrs McTernan would keep them chatting and have everything tidy by the time I arrived. I was surrounded by pubs; one was almost next door, another was 30 yards further up, and another up about 100 yards from the surgery. All could see whether my car was at the surgery or not, so all they had to do was walk out into the street to see if the doctor had arrived, finish their drink and come down to the waiting room.

After closing the surgery I frequently found a drink had been left in some of the pubs as a present for me. One of the differences between Gortin and Belcoo was that in Gortin the doctor who took a drink was frowned upon, whereas in Belcoo he was considered to be one of the people if he would stand up to the counter and take a drink.

Dr Hamilton had never been a drinking man; although he enjoyed a drink with a medical friend in private, he was not a man to go into a pub and converse with the locals. Dr Hawkins had no such reservations. The first time I stood in for him and did a surgery in Glenlevin I was quite busy, but when the patients were all seen I went into Johnny Mickey Ruadh's bar, which was attached to the dispensary, to have a bottle of stout. I found a line of whiskeys sitting on the bar waiting and I didn't know they were for me. I asked for a bottle of stout and Johnny asked me, did I want to finish these first? When I asked, 'Where did these come from?' he said, 'Oh, the patients left them for you – they always do that for Doctor Hawkins.'

What could I do, refuse them and insult the patrons who were still in the bar? All I could do was drink them. I watered them well and got into great conversation with the donors, Johnny, his wife and family and had one whale of an evening. By the time I had most of them finished it was time to eat and I admitted to Johnny that I felt under the weather. Actually, I was plastered. Mrs Johnny got me into the kitchen, put up a mixed grill and plenty of home-made soda bread, which soaked up a lot of the whiskey before it got absorbed. When I was fit to walk to the car alone I was considered sober enough to drive home down the long hill into Blacklion. I reported in to Mrs Hawkins that I had done the surgery and seen to everybody who needed it, including a few house calls. She said, 'Yerra, ye got out of there more sober than Bill comes, so they must have watered your whiskey.'

As I got to know Bill Hawkins better I would sometimes drop by the dispensary when he was holding court and share some of this whiskey with him. They would be sitting on the bar, lined up, and he would just push one towards me when he took one himself, neither of us paying for anything, but I never really saw him obviously drunk. I am sure Maisie, his wife, would see drunkenness on him more easily than I. He sent me home under the weather on several occasions when he seemed to me to be stone-cold sober.

About 1955, one evening I went into Philip Dolan's pub to get petrol and there was a big hearty gentleman at the counter talking to Philip. I told Philip I needed petrol, so he came out and filled the tank. He said, 'There's a fella in there at the bar called McCorry who will bullshit you. He retired from the Civic Guards.'

We returned to the bar and he introduced me to Johnty McCorry. These policemen all had a vast knowledge of what was going on all over Ireland, not only in places like Blacklion. He said, 'Where are you from?'

I said, 'I'm from Dublin.'

He asked, 'Where in Dublin?'

I said, 'Terenure.'

'Ah,' he said, 'I was in Tallaght, I was a Guard there. You wouldn't be anything to do with a Doctor McCann from Terenure?'

I replied, 'I'm his son.'

'Ah,' he said, 'I'll have to buy you a drink. Doctor Sean McCann used to treat all us Guards and never charged us a penny. We all voted that he should be the Guards' doctor but the wrong political party was in power at the time and Sean Lavin got the job.' Dr Sean Lavin was a great athlete, he won prizes all over the world for running.

Anyway, from then on, Johnty and I were friends. He could start at ten o'clock in the morning and keep going until ten at night telling stories about when he was in 'the Depot' (the police academy in Dublin). He had a fantastic sense of humour. I doubt if I heard any of his stories twice. I was always glad to see him. He knew Philip didn't like him but that didn't stop him from going into Philip's bar and saying the very things that he knew Philip hated to hear. He'd wink at me and he'd say, 'When I was in the Depot...' and this was like a red rag to a bull for Philip, who would look up at the ceiling as much as to say, 'Another Depot story.' Johnty was one of these people who are good at everything. He was a great shot with a shotgun and I noticed during the few times I went out shooting with him he never aimed at anything but he hit it. I was not so lucky. I never went shooting enough to ever become good at it.

Johnty and I went fishing and we never went out on the lakes that he did not come back with at least a dozen fish. About 3 miles away from Blacklion there was a lake up in the hills, called Garraway Lake, which was owned by his uncle. We could go fishing there at any time and they had a boat on the lake. I had never fished since I was a child fishing with worms, and never caught anything. Johnty decided he was going to make a fisherman out of me. We went to Bertie's hardware store next door to Philip's pub and he got Bertie to bring out all the flies and he picked the ones we were going to use.

Two days later we got organized. We had lines, rods, reels, the whole thing. We got into my car, as he didn't have one at that time. After we got up to the lake he got out the boat and rowed us out into the middle. He showed me how to make out a line with three flies and in no time he had caught three fish. I caught nothing. Before the day was over, Johnty had caught a dozen fish and I still had nothing. We went there frequently and I never caught a fish. He always did most of the rowing and caught all the fish.

Sometimes his sister would fry the fish in her cottage by the lake and sometimes we'd drive back to Philip's pub and he or Johnty would fry them in the kitchen after closing time. We would eat them at the bar, which Philip would cover with newspapers and plates, in what he called the 'Shelbourne Night'. This was after the Shelbourne Hotel in Dublin. Whenever he knew we were going fishing he'd say, 'Are we going to have a Shelbourne Night?' This was to find out if he was going to get a slice of the action.

One fair day we arrived back in Philip's with fish and the bar was full and so was Philip. There was no question of a 'Shelbourne'. We had about 20 trout and they were big ones. We left a few for Philip and went back to Johnty's home, where his sister, who lived with his mother, fried them and we had a really good meal with a dozen stouts and it was a fun evening.

The following morning after I closed the surgery I decided to go over to Blacklion with Master Cox, whom I had met outside. Master Cox was a retired schoolteacher who used to teach in Holywell School outside Belcoo. He was between 65 and 70 years old. Every day he had a ritual; he went down to Belcoo, bought a newspaper, went into one of the pubs, either P. Mickey's, McGuire's or P. Rosey's. He had a whiskey or a stout and then walked to Blacklion, where he discussed with Philip Dolan the likely horses for that day. He made some bets, which were picked up by a bus driver who went into Enniskillen daily and laid bets with a bookie there.

This day I came out of my surgery and Master Cox was walking by. He invited me to go to Blacklion to have a drink. I got him into my car and we drove over to Philip. When we went in, Philip was red-faced and furious. Really bad humour, a 'bad story' all over the place. Philip was full. Anyway, we ordered our drinks and finally found out what had occurred with Philip. As it was a fair day, Phil had got good and high the night before and when he had emptied the bar, he brought his fish into the back and fried them. As they were frying, he laid his newspapers on the kitchen table and when they were done, he put the fish down and ate them (he probably drank whiskey with them); but there was something that was Philip's secret until that day. He really didn't enjoy eating with his teeth in. He had false teeth, top and bottom, so he had taken the teeth out and left them beside the plate while he was eating. His meal finished, he rolled everything up in the newspapers and put it in the turf fire which he always kept going in the kitchen. He went off to bed and in the morning he reached out to get his teeth. No teeth! The teeth had gone with the fishbones into the fire. He had to go away and get a new set, top and bottom. There was no way this could be kept a secret and Philip took a lot of 'chopper' jokes for a long time after that.

The next time we brought fish to Philip, Johnty said, 'I think Philip you'd better give me your teeth to bring home or they won't be safe.' Philip was not amused. 'Depot', as he called Johnty, was not the one to amuse him. The madder Philip got the funnier and the more enjoyable Johnty found the situation.

One evening we went into Philip's and Johnty said, 'This should be good weather for fishing.' Apparently good weather for fishing was a breezy day without too much sun, even rainy weather was good, but a sunny day was not good, not on Johnty's lake, according to him. Philip heard our plans to get out the following morning before daybreak, arrive at the lake before sunrise and get in a good morning's fishing. It would be a Saturday because I was not going to open my surgery.

It was arranged that I would pick up Philip and drive to Johnty's and pick him up and we would all go to the lake. The following morning I was there bright and early, just before dawn, and I had my doubts if I would be able to get Philip out of bed because his house was three storeys high and I didn't think he would hear me knocking at his door. However, when I got there, Philip was sleepy and also under the weather. He knew that we would not be able to waken him, so he had stayed in his car all night. He was wearing a trenchcoat and in every pocket he had a flat bottle of whiskey, a 'naggin' as they called it in those days. He gave each of us a naggin when we got to Johnty's place.

We got the fishing rods into the car and off we went to the lake, where we got Philip into the boat. He got all tangled up in his fishing line, he got the hooks in his clothes and finally gave up. He put it all away and sat in the boat while we fished. Johnty caught the fish and I think I caught one. By lunchtime Philip had had enough and we had all had enough because we had been drinking Philip's naggins. We headed back to Philip's with the fish and ate them in his kitchen on the usual newspaper. That was the last time we went fishing with Philip. He never brought up the subject again or gave any indication that he was inclined to fish or join us early in the morning or at any time of the day.

I happened to meet Major Nixon one day in the avenue at his home and mentioned our fishing escapades up in the Garraway Lake. He told me he had a very good fishing lake up in Boho on his land which he hadn't fished in years because he hadn't been able. He told me I could go up there and fish any time I wished – just tell his land steward who lived on the lake that we had his permission. There was a boat, oars, everything there; all we needed to take was our fishing tackle. Shortly after that Johnty and I went up there and fished. We could hardly bring them in quick enough.

It was a windy day with a nice ripple on the lake and we must have caught about 30 nice trout. We dropped off ten of them for Major Nixon, for which he was very grateful and left us carte blanche to go and fish there any time we wished. We did return but never caught anything again, not one fish. They probably hadn't seen a fisherman for so long they were just asking to be caught the first time.

What we did not know was that Major Nixon had told one of his friends about our fantastic catch. Some years later, when Major Nixon was dead and this friend bought his house and we got to know him well, he told us that he had gone up with an 'otter' and cleaned the lake out. An otter is a device which, when you row or propel a boat along you let the otter out of the side of the boat and it floats parallel to the boat. It is weighted in such a way that as the boat moves it moves on – the same principle as a kite – away from the boat. Lines a foot apart attached to the line holding the otter have bait on them. The result is 12 hooks are moving forward with bait on them and they catch many fish. So every time he took 10 to 12 fish when he got to the end of the lake. He would then rebait the hooks and make another run. Using an electric motor, he had soon caught most of the fish in the lake.

He got something like 500 fish, which he sold to the local hotels, so no wonder Johnty and I never caught another fish. I am sure the Major would have been furious had he known. We certainly were. Davy was a hearty, funny man and thought this was an hilarious joke on the Major. The Major was a humourless crank but he had been good to me and I wouldn't have dreamed of doing anything like that to him for any reason.

We found living in the flat to be very pleasant. The Major and his daughter, who came to visit once in a while from England, would send the gardener up with fresh vegetables occasionally to keep the friendship going but I never became close to the Nixons as there was no way one could warm up to him. He kept himself at a distance, as did his English wife.

After some months the Major used his influence with a friend of his who had land near Belcoo and had built a duplex which he usually rented to policemen. A policeman had left one of the homes in the duplex and I accepted it. It was a two-storey with three upstairs bedrooms, a sitting room and kitchen downstairs, both very large, and a bathroom for which the water had to be pumped from a pump outside the house. Had I known as much as I know now, I should have had an electric pump installed. The dark old range we replaced by a Raeburn stove. This heated water as well as being a wonderful cooking stove. We installed a fridge, so we were again in luxury. A large garden was attached to it with front flower garden and large lawn around the side. In the house next door was Mr Raesdale, a British Customs officer who ran the border operation on the northern side of the border. He and his wife were very pleasant neighbours and they had two nice children who went to school in Enniskillen by bus.

Now that we had a house with three upstairs rooms there was room to hire a maid, who slept in the small room and the children in one of the larger rooms. I now had a lock-up surgery and I made sure that nobody but Mrs McTernan and I entered it, and I almost had to confide in her that Gloria could not come up and borrow the key and get in.

Nevertheless, Gloria on two occasions did get access by telling Mrs McTernan that there was an emergency and that another doctor was covering for me.

4

Gathering Storms

I renewed acquaintance with Dr Curran, who had a practice in Kinawley on the border of Swanlibar and Fermanagh, 12 miles away. We covered for each other and our practices were very similar. We developed a routine of playing golf in Enniskillen Golf Club and in Belturbet Golf Club, all within reasonable distance, and on weekends we could go to Bundoran, where I had wrecked the car. There was a very good golf course there also.

In 1956 a jolly Irish priest was appointed to the Blacklion Parish called Killinagh. Father Walter McGrath had been in the United States and had recently returned because of his mother's poor health. She accompanied him to Killinagh and was a very pleasant lady but up in years. She became my patient and Father Walter became my friend. On our trips to Bundoran Dr Curran and I would go with Father Walter, who had a big Wolsey car, and it was a luxurious way to travel.

Father Walter had been on the west coast of the United States, mostly in Los Angeles and the south, and he had spent some time in Montana and Wyoming. While in California he had been in San Diego, which he had loved and about which he told us lots of interesting stories. He was an excellent golfer, indicating that he did not spend all his time praying when he was in the United States.

On our Sundays in Bundoran, Gloria came together with Dr Curran's wife and we would leave them on the beach with the children. Although Martha didn't drink seriously, Gloria could somehow manage to get somewhere where they could have a drink and by the time we got back from the golf she would usually be pretty merry. Eventually I had to confide in Dr Curran about Gloria's problems. I also had to tell the chemist in Enniskillen from whom I got most of my medications that she was not to have any medication or get access to the back of his shop – and I had to tell him the reason for this.

About 1956 Gloria was again pregnant and I had her visit Dr Smith, who had delivered Keevsa. She would take the car and drive to Enniskillen on her own and sometimes she would bring the children with her. On one of these occasions I got a phone call from the police to say that Gloria had been stopped for passing a car on the wrong side. They said they would keep her until she was in a fit condition to drive, indicating that she was intoxicated. We had only one car so all I could do was to wait until the police got her home. They very obligingly sent a policeman to drive her home and I drove him back to Enniskillen.

When Gloria was about six months pregnant I came home one evening to find her stuporous in bed – the result of a combination of alcohol and morphine. I found a vial of morphine under her pillow. She had been to see Dr Smith and apparently gone through his desk when he was out of the room. I could think of no other way she could have obtained it.

When I confronted her the following morning she denied it and did not know how the vial got under her pillow. I had to tell Dr Smith the problem and he told me that he would take precautions in future. I am sorry to say he didn't, and twice prior to her delivery I found morphine and her condition showing evidence that she had used it. She did not get any more abscesses so I presume that the syringes she was using were either stolen out of my car or out of Dr Curran's car, where we kept them sterile. There was also the possibility that she got them from Dr Smith's surgery.

About a month prior to her delivery I drove her to Fintona to see her parents. I had been up the night before on a maternity case, on a delivery, and I was tired. I asked her to drive the car home. I noticed at one stage that she was unsteady and driving pretty erratically. I said we should pull off the road and I would have a nap and then I would drive the rest of the way. We pulled off the road and the next thing I woke up and the car was upside down in a ditch beside a hedge. Apparently Gloria had taken it upon herself to drive on and there was some ice. She skidded on the ice and the car was wedged in the ditch. I was not driving, I was in the passenger seat, so I was able to climb out the window. It was a Volkswagen and I could smell petrol. I was afraid it might go on fire and I tried to get her out but I couldn't. She was jammed behind the steering wheel. In a Volkswagen when you got into a situation like that the seat frequently jumped forward and it was impossible to get out from behind it. I stopped a passing car and got the local garage to come and get her out. They came with a tractor and pulled the car out. It was badly wrecked and again I was without a car for about six weeks. I was back to motorcycles.

When the baby was due the local nurse was called and the delivery was to be at home. Dr Smith was called but he was not available. His sister said that he would be delayed but he would come as soon as he could.

The baby was stillborn. It was hard to say whether it was the result of drugs, turning the car over or a combination of both.

Garvan and Keevsa were now going to school. This was 1957 and there was no improvement whatsoever in Gloria's addiction and behaviour.

I could see that there was little future in remaining in this practice and as I was unlikely ever to get an equally good practice in Northern Ireland, I began to look at overseas jobs in the *British Medical Journal*.

I applied for a position in the New Zealand Navy. If I succeeded in obtaining it, I could have my family moved to New Zealand free, spend ten years with the navy and have a pension. I went to London to be interviewed and have a medical examination but I failed the medical because of hypertension. I also felt that I did not do well in the interview because of the interviewing doctor asking me why I did not join the Royal Navy, which could give me equally good benefits. I could not tell him that I had to get Gloria as far away as possible from Ireland and the environment. I thought if I could get to New Zealand there would be some chance of keeping her away from medications in a strange country.

Shortly after the trip to London one of my patients had to go to court, having been beaten up by some of his local neighbours. He was a young man who was slightly retarded and had been the butt of some rustic humour of some of his neighbours. Anyway, he was injured and could no longer help his father on their small farm. I went to court to give evidence that he could no longer do heavy farm work because of his back injury. Because I was passing their house on the way to court, I gave him, his father and two witnesses a ride. The boy won the case, with compensation.

Driving home, we came to a turn in the road, halfway between Enniskillen and Belcoo, where there were new screenings on the road. This meant that new gravel had been spread on the road and there was tar in the middle but the sides were not tarred. When we came to this long curve I got into a skid, the back of the car got into the screenings on the left side of the road, slid around and when it came to the hard surface again it caught, and the car rolled over. The young man, who was sitting next to me, was thrown around inside the car and when it came upright there was a bus coming in the opposite direction and his door hit the bus. We were all badly shaken. I broke three ribs. The car was totalled. The three men in the back seemed to be all right. I was badly shaken and shocked, and I and the young boy were taken to hospital in Enniskillen. He was found to have fractured the base of his skull and died that night.

After two days in hospital I left and went to Waterford to spend some time with my brother Kevin, who came to pick me up and to get over the disaster. A locum covered my practice. When I claimed insurance the company refused to pay because they said there should not have been three people in the back of the car. The only thing I could do was to buy a cheap car and get my insurance in the Republic and run it back and forth across the border.

Finally, the Customs people in the North got wise to the fact that I was driving a southern car and refused to let it cross the border. I was back to bicycles. I could not get insurance for a motorcycle so I had to cycle and use taxis.

Johnty McCorry was of inestimable help because he had at this stage bought a car and was running it as a taxi. He could drive me into Northern Ireland if I met him in the Republic. It was a very complicated way of getting around and running a practice and I knew that the time had come and I was definitely at an end.

The garage man, a friend of mine, in Omagh, Co. Tyrone, bought the remains of my Volkswagen, which was a beautiful car before the wreck as I had only had it for about three months. He sold me a cheap old Ford Anglia and registered it and insured it in his name, John James. This was quite illegal but we did not get caught. I had also practically given him the Volkswagen wreck for a song but he had a way of disposing of the parts as he was in the used car business.

I got out the *British Medical Journal* again and began to answer the advertisements.

I did not want to work in England or the British Isles because of Gloria. I knew that she would ruin me again if I got into another practice, even into an assistantship. I would have to acquaint my employer with her problems and that would be the end of my job.

5

Flight to Freedom

One morning in 1959, about September, I got a letter with a foreign postmark and stamp and hieroglyphics on the envelope. When I opened it it was from a doctor in Iran, with a company called Amman & Whitney of New York and The Plan Organization, which was the company building roads in that country. They requested a curriculum vitae and some references, which I promptly got, including Father Walter and the local schoolteachers and Dr Curran and Dr Quinn. They all gave me glowing references.

Dr Flamank was the doctor who had written to me from Iran and he made an appointment to meet me in Dublin at the end of September to discuss the proposition of employment in Iran. Vincent McGovern volunteered to drive me up to the interview and he left me outside the Gresham Hotel in Dublin. I brought Gloria along, both to keep her out of trouble at home and to have the doctor meet her and to know what kind of a family we were.

Inside the hotel I paged Dr Flamank and he met me in the bar and we sat down and had a drink. He was charming, had a good sense of humour and we got on very well indeed. He had his wife with him and we sat and had several more drinks and I told him about the kind of practice I had and that the future for me in Northern Ireland was poor, including the fact that I wasn't 'digging with the right foot', which meant that I was the wrong religion. He took all this down and was very interested and before I left I had a job.

He had me sign a form of agreement and told me that it would probably be December before I could get there. He gave me all the instructions on how to get visas and passport etc. to immigrate into Iran. Whatever it cost, I was to let him know and he would forward expenses, travel money and everything else.

In two weeks I was in the Iranian Embassy in London. I spent a couple of days in London and did all the work necessary to get a passport, immigration visas etc. I then had to go back to Dublin to get an Irish passport and in four weeks I was ready to move.

I resigned from my practice by writing to Belfast and gave them a month's notice. All my patients were notified that I had given up practice and to advise them to get another doctor. Unfortunately, the patients south of the border thought I would not see them either and the practice just folded. Nobody at all came near me from then on.

I told Vincent McGovern my predicament and that my money had suddenly stopped. He said not to worry he would employ me driving cars from the west of Ireland to Enniskillen. So every week we made one or two trips to Co. Mayo, Co. Galway, Co. Clare and Sligo buying cars. New cars were available in the Republic but they were not available in Northern Ireland. These used cars were now being allowed to be brought across the border and Vincent had a licence to do this. Twice a week we would go to places like Co. Mayo, places you never heard of, buying cars from people who were buying new cars. Four of us would go, with Johnty McCorry driving us on some trips, and we would come back with three cars plus the car we went in. Some of our drivers were local policemen.

They were great jaunts indeed. We would arrive in the town, go around, look at the cars, buy them for cash and drive home. We stopped in pubs in towns I had never seen before and will never see again, but Johnty or the policemen with us or somebody knew somebody in every one of them.

If I had not had so many arrangements made, I seriously thought that I would have gone into this business full-time. Although Vincent was paying very generously I was not sure if he was not carrying me on his back. I did not like to ask any of the others how much he paid them.

Vincent arranged a big send-off party for me nearer to the time of my departure. I was to be in Iran on 21 December 1959. I would have to go before Christmas, and leaving Gloria and the kids and everyone at home was very sad.

The night of the party the town of Blacklion was a riot. The pubs were packed, every one of them, and every pub I went into I got a drink and spent nothing. There was a collection made and I was presented with a silver watch, a Rolex engraved with my name and the dates I had come and left. Their gratitude and anything that they could fit on the back was engraved on it. People came from as far away as Gortin and Enniskillen, Carrickmore and Trillick. People I never knew, knew me. Everyone that I had ever visited in their house, people that I had never charged, contributed generously.

There was one big problem that nearly stalled everything. I could not get a passport until I got letters from my banks that I was clear of debt. My overdraft at this stage was £1,500. There was no way I could rustle up the money, but Bertie Armstrong and a Mr Carson, who owned a quarry between Enniskillen and Belcoo, came to my rescue. I had approached them and asked them if they could help. Between them they put up the difference that was necessary to clear my overdraft, believing my promise that I would pay them back as soon as I got overseas. As it happened I was able to get an advance when I got to Iran and pay them in three months.

Our farewells at the barrier at the Dublin airport were not tearful but close to it. The children did not realize what was happening and Gloria and I had had a few drinks at the bar so we were able to console ourselves that it was only going to be a two-year separation. I was sad because I still loved her. Vincent was as sad as anybody else because our friendship had become very close and he had proven himself an exceptional friend by giving me every assistance. He promised to look after Gloria and the children and would see that they had no financial difficulties until I got on my feet. I had left Gloria as much money as I could, everything I had, except £25 which I thought I might need for the trip. I had cut it pretty fine because when I caught the last plane out of London for Teheran I had £5 in my wallet and small change.

I spent about two days in London in a boarding house not far from the London Airport terminal. From there I visited the Iranian Consulate to get my visa and passport finalized and to show evidence that I was a physician and that I had employment when I arrived in Iran. I had Dr Flamank's literature and copies of everything needed, as he had known what I would have to have.

The first part of the flight on BOAC was to Frankfurt. The duty-free shop there was staggering, and although I didn't have anything to spend I nearly missed the plane because I couldn't hear myself being paged in it. Anyway, when I got to the plane it was waiting for me. The next stop was Damascus and it was night. The vendors in the airport selling carpets and all kinds of radios, electronics, cameras etc., were very interesting to me indeed. They were all speaking English which left me unprepared for what I was going to experience in Teheran.

I arrived in Teheran at dawn and, not knowing what to expect, I was going to be surprised anyway. I had never seen anything so drab and brown as we came in. The plane circled the airport and I could see the undulating hills, all brown. There was no heather or green here. It was 21 December and winter. When I finally got through the airport the officials could speak English and could understand me. I had no carry-on luggage because I had no carry-on bag. I had no knowledge of the 'niceties' of travel and all I had in my pockets were my papers, my passport and my ticket. I asked a man outside in the street how I could get to Teheran. He looked at me blankly and then, thinking he might be deaf, I spoke louder and he walked away. I hauled my two bags into the airport again, expecting to be met by somebody because they knew I was coming. I learned later that they had thought I was arriving the previous day, and when I didn't turn up they were not going to come every day and see if I was on the plane.

I thought I would call Amman & Whitney's office to see what was going on and I took a telephone directory, but there was no English anywhere – it was all in Farsi. I went to a telephone and I had no coinage to fit. This was the first experience I had ever had of being somewhere where English was not spoken. I began to feel a slight panic and I thought I would buy some cigarettes to get change but they would not take my money. I had sterling only. The situation was one that I had never even imagined could happen. Finally, I went to the bookshop and there was a lady behind the counter. I spoke to her and discovered she could speak good English. I told her of my predicament and she said she would call Amman & Whitney. I had the number on the letters I had received from Dr Flamank. She finally got through to the office and gave me the telephone. I spoke to a very nice lady with an English accent who reassured me that she would send out Dr Tim to pick me up in one of the company's cars. I stood outside the airport waiting. There were not many people around so I put my bags down and wandered up and down.

After about 20 minutes a car pulled up and a man got out whom I recognized. He was Tim Counihan who had been my student at St Vincent's Hospital in Dublin and was a medical student when I left so I had not seen him in ten years. Was he glad to see me and was I glad to see him. We had so much to talk about. I had so many questions to ask, and so had he. I didn't know how he didn't know it was I who was coming, but he was surprised. He said had he known it was me, he would have been out there waiting for every plane from London.

We got to the Amman & Whitney office and I was introduced to a very beautiful English lady with an Irish name, Betty Cahail. Tim told me, 'If you want anything, ask Betty. Betty runs this place and she knows everything', and how right he was. I was later to find that Betty could conjure up food, drink, emergency equipment, anything that was needed down the road or in the city.

Tim brought me over to the Jam Hotel almost directly across the street, about 100 yards west of the office. I had a beautiful room, bathroom attached, air-conditioning and everything that one could ask for. Having dumped my stuff Tim's first idea was, 'Let's have a drink.' We had a drink down in the bar in the hotel but Tim said it was too expensive, so he brought me around the block to a *pension* where there was a bar. It reminded me of a place in Dublin called Dolly Fawcett's, which was a house of ill repute. When I mentioned this to Tim, he laughed and said, 'You mightn't be far wrong, but this place is a bit better class than Dolly Fawcett's was.' He knew Dolly's as well as I did. Every medical student in

Dublin knew Dolly's where you could get a drink at any hour of the night as long as you had enough money to pay the extra.

After a couple of Iranian beers, mixed with a little vodka, we were both in great shape and headed back to the office, where I met Dr Flamank and Mr Sherman. The latter was the chief of the whole operation. I felt like the long-lost son. There were other gentlemen there, male nurses, two of them. Each doctor was to have a male nurse with him in his hospital.

The Shah had been married the day before, this being 21 December 1959. All anyone could speak about was the wedding and the Shah's bride driving past the office and waving to everyone. While I was crossing the street it was fortunate that I had Tim with me as I looked the wrong way, unaware that everyone was driving on the right side of the road and not the left as in Britain and Ireland. I stepped off the kerb, looked the other way, and nearly got hit by a taxi, which swerved to avoid me. The streets were broad and there were not many high-rises but quite an amount of building projects going on. High-rises were about to be built.

I could not get over the taxis. For 10 rials, which was about sixpence in my money, you could go anywhere in the city. Nobody walked. There were buses, but they were always so full up they didn't stop at every stop and anyway you couldn't read the destination written in Farsi. Everything was in Farsi. The car numbers were written in figures I couldn't understand but Tim and the other two male nurses educated me and were full of knowledge about what the figures meant.

That night we went to the Shu Café and brought Betty. She knew her way around and she was great fun. She took a lot of ragging from the boys and she could rag them back. There was a show on and a lady wrestled with an alligator and a snake. A contortionist got up on stage and I thought he would break his own neck. It was all terribly new, interesting and exciting and a completely different world. The people looked so different – to me they were all 'foreigners' – and many men had moustaches.

I hardly slept that night at all, even though I was full of booze. The following morning I was up early to see what was going on. We hung around the office a lot and I had changed my money into

Iranian money but I was running short. Tim said, 'There is no problem, tell Betty.' Betty got me an advance and I thought I would never see a poor day again. Although I hadn't done any work the money was forthcoming any time I needed it. When I thought back on how difficult it was getting money in Ireland and how much trouble I had getting my bank overdraft cleared, it began to dawn on me that I had not left Ireland half soon enough.

Dr Flamank told me that when I was in London he had tried to get in touch with me to tell me not to come yet, that my hospital was not ready and I could have really stayed in Ireland for Christmas and come in the New Year, but it was too late now.

The second night after I arrived there was a party in Mr Sherman's home, a cocktail party. Everyone was introduced to everyone else. There were Greeks, Scotsmen, two Irishmen and Americans galore. Mrs Sherman was a charming hostess and there was enough food to feed an army.

When the party was over we walked back to the Jam Hotel as it was not a great distance. We had some engineers with us, Germans, Dr French and Tim and I. Tim was staying in the *pension*. He left me at the Jam Hotel and I tumbled into bed. It was great to have a shower and a bath, so I could bath at night and shower in the morning. It was probably the food but I felt remarkably well in spite of all the booze we had had at the Shermans'.

There was nowhere to go but to the office, and of course Sunday came around and we were all looking for somewhere to go to church. I was still a practising Catholic and a lot of the engineers were also, so they brought me to a church around the corner. Sunday is a weekday in Iran because the Moslem sabbath is on Friday and people had to take time off to get to church if they were going to practise their religion diligently.

On Christmas Day Dr Flamank had us over and played records of Christmas carols and a lot of sentimental music, which made us all very sad, especially Bob Loughman, one of the nurses. Every time he heard 'Should Auld Acquaintance be Forgot' he wept. He wept copiously that night, as I did myself, wondering if the toys and presents I had left for the children had been delivered. Some of the boys had radios and could get the BBC. We were three and a half hours ahead of Greenwich Mean Time, so we listened to the 8 o'clock news at 11.30 p.m.

Finally, Dr Flamank had to do something about all these doctors and nurses, so he got us tickets to 'go down the line' as they called the road project. He sent us to a place called Pol-i-doktar. We were put on a train on Boxing Day in Teheran which left town at about 4.00 p.m., and we were expected to arrive in Andimeshk the following morning, probably about 8.00 a.m.

There was a buffet car on the train and we could have some Iranian bread, which was unleavened, and rice and eggs. The eggs were almost raw but they broke them on top of the rice. I was so hungry that I ate the whole thing, and I got to like Iranian bread, which was like chewing a piece of leather, but it was food. The train had roll-out beds which you folded out, and the seats turned into a bed when the porter came in and changed them. I was travelling with Bob Loughman, the male nurse, in one carriage and there was a man across from us coughing. He coughed all night. Bob thought he probably had TB and would infect us, but I knew I was immune to TB because I had been checked as a medical student. Bob was a delicate kind of chap in his own estimation and very conscious of his health. Finally, the train stopped at Andimeshk and we got out with our goods and chattels. We were met there by somebody from Amman & Whitney who got us a taxi and sent us off to Pol-i-doktar.

The taxi had to travel along a paved road for the first 5 or 6 miles, maybe 10. It seemed like 100. There were enormous potholes which the driver had to avoid. He'd drive along and there would be a pothole and he would move to the other side of the road. It was just absolutely unbelievable. This was why the hospitals had been built along the road between Teheran and the south of Iran. A road had been built during the war to get munitions into the back door of Russia to fight the Germans. It had been built quickly by the British and the Americans just to get the tanks and munitions, trucks etc. in from the Gulf of Iran. After years of neglect and no upkeep, the road had practically become non-existent. It would have been better if it had not been paved at all because the potholes were deep and sharp. Eventually we got on to a rough road which had not been paved and could make good time. We arrived in Pol-i-doktar to meet the engineers and Dr Butler, who had been one of the first doctors in the system. Hospitality was great and we met Betty's boyfriend, an engineer called Tom. We listened to record players, music of all descriptions, drank and ate well. We were to all intents and purposes to replace Dr Butler. He took the taxi we had arrived in and went back to Teheran.

The following day I had my first patient, who had spilt petrol and been burned. He was brought to the hospital, blistered from head to foot. His clothes were burned and even the threads in his shoes had been burned so that the soles came off. The people who brought him in on a stretcher were hilariously enjoying this as they thought it was the funniest thing they had ever seen. Apparently when he was burning they had laughed and danced around. I couldn't believe it. We had an ambulance and there was no way we could treat him in our hospital so he had to be brought to Hamadan. I had no idea how far it was or how long it would take to get there.

This was my first experience of driving through the heartland, apart from the trip up from Andimeshk. This was something different. It was a mountainous road and it had been cut out of the side of a mountain. The closest thing I could compare it to was a fly walking along a picture rail, the old-fashioned kind. It was a sheer drop down to our left and a sheer rock rising to the right. I sat in front beside the driver, and the nurse, Mr White, sat behind with the patient. The road was still being built and every so often there were graders, diggers, cranes and all kinds of machinery, but the climb was steady. Every few miles our ears would click; it was very high and the altitude was increasing. On the way the nurse and I decided we needed to empty our bladders, so the driver stopped and I got out of the door on my side. That was a mistake. I was soon up to my knees in mud, wet mucky mud. I had gone so far that I had to walk around the ambulance to get back to solid road. When I got in again the mud dried and became stiff and hard. It was a most uncomfortable trip.

The first place we arrived at was Khorramabad. This was where Tim had his hospital, and he looked after us while we were there. He gave us a meal and some whiskey to warm us up. It was getting colder as the altitude increased. The driver said we should not stop after that. We kept going – it seemed to have been about 24 hours, a confusion in time because I did not know where I was just that it was either night or day. There was no greenery, only rock and brown hills and the most monotonous country one could imagine. It was like being on the moon.

At night it was extremely dangerous but at least we were on the side of the road where the rock rose up. When we met a car or truck, our driver would put out his lights and the other driver would put out his. This alternating lights on and lights off continued until one passed the other. It would be very dangerous for the traffic going the other way because if they slipped off to the right they were over the precipice and that was it. Further along, however, the mountains were on the other side and we had the precipice to our right so what was sauce for the goose was also sauce for the gander. I was always afraid of driving at night in Iran because of this alternate flashing of the lights, but never so much so as between Pol-i-doktar and Hamadan. Finally, the second night out we arrived in Hamadan at about two in the morning. There was nobody about, but the ambulance man, who could speak Farsi, asked a policeman where the hospital was.

When we got there I couldn't believe what I saw. Inside the door there were patients lying on mattresses on the cement floor next to each other with no space between them. When our patient was brought in one of the attendants chased one of the patients out of his bed and put our patient in it. The patient would not be seen by a doctor until the following day but at least we had enough morphine to keep giving it to him whenever he showed signs of pain. This was about every three hours and this was what had been keeping him alive until we had got him there. Nobody seemed to have any pity at all for the poor man who was burned. I don't know how he survived.

The trip back to Pol-i-doktar was more relaxed. There was no hurry and we stopped at various *chai-khanas*, or teahouses, along the way and had tea with a lot of sugar in it, and we smoked. The ambulance we were using was a Volkswagen, well equipped and very comfortable. We had three or four of them, supposedly one to each hospital, and that was our transport going shopping or bringing patients from one place to another.

Mr White persuaded the driver to let him drive for a while, which the driver reluctantly did. He turned over the wheel and the three of us sat in the front seat which was a wide bench.

We came to a town called Burujird, which was in a fairly flat area, and while driving through it we found that there must have been a fair or a market or something because there were a lot of people in the streets, many of them with donkeys and the donkeys were laden with what resembled creels that they use in Ireland. On top of one of these loaded donkeys was a big pregnant woman. Something distracted Mr White, and the lady's donkey swung out in front of him. He hit it with the front of the ambulance and she fell off her perch. There was instant panic and shouting and gathering around. People were shouting at Mr White and shouting at the ambulance driver who was the only one who could speak Farsi. The woman did not seem much the worse for wear. She would not get up, however, and stayed lying on the ground. It was a nice dry sunny day and the ground was dusty but not dirty. Next the police arrived and the poor driver was very busy interpreting. Because Mr White did not have a driving licence he was immediately in trouble. He was arrested and put in jail. The driver had to call Teheran, which took hours to do, and get through to the main office to arrange for an attorney etc.

We could not get Mr White out of jail so we decided to spend the night in town in the hotel, such as it was. It was very primitive but there was a restaurant and we were able to eat and take some food over to Mr White in jail. Dr Flamank got in touch with us from Teheran and there was hell to pay up there. He flew down to Andimeshk, where a company jeep brought him to Burujird, where we were. There he got in touch with a local lawyer. Dr Flamank had brought money with him, and when a sufficient amount had been agreed upon as to how much the woman and her husband should get, we were free to leave.

We all got driving licences after that because a driver was not always available and having a driver on the premises meant he had to be housed etc. – one driver even insisted on having his family with him in Avej when I was there.

We got back to Pol-i-doktar and I finished out my two weeks' coverage for Dr Butler. When he returned, Dr Flamank came down with him and transported me and Mr Bob Loughman, the male nurse, back to a hospital further up the line north of Hamadan to a place called Avej. This was where I was to spend the remainder of my time in Iran.

6

Life in Avej

On the journey from Pol-i-doktar to Avej, with Dr Flamank driving the ambulance, we ran into trouble. We got into a garage in Khorramabad, where we spent the night. It was dark when we arrived and the ambulance was pulled into an examination pit to be checked the next morning. Bob Loughman, getting out of the ambulance, didn't know that the pit extended in front of the ambulance. He tried to step across in front and fell into it. He complained of pains in his head and neck but by the following morning he seemed to be all right, although his pains persisted. The ambulance was fixed and the drive to Avej was completed that day.

The Avej camp was about 7 miles south of Avej on the Hamadan road. Dr Flamank introduced us to the contractor, Carlos, who had a big home, like a ranch house. He was very hospitable and we had a very nice meal. Carlos was Italian, and he produced an enormous salad, spaghetti and dessert. Beds had been set up in the engineers' building, in which the front room was an office and rooms at the back had been converted into bedrooms. There was a hot shower and bathroom so we all got up the next morning, showered, dressed and had breakfast with Carlos. Dr Flamank packed his ambulance and left, promising to send it back with a driver.

The engineers' office had been set up as a dispensary and was well equipped with medications and instruments, emergency sets for stitching, suturing and anything that might turn up unexpectedly. There was really nothing to do as there were no patients. Mr Loughman and I walked around the camp and explored the surrounding countryside. There were lanes and side roads but the main road was still under construction and very rough and muddy. I had my medical books, so I had something to read. The area engineer arrived about ten in the morning from Hamadan, where he resided in the Bou Ali Hotel. As we had no transport and nothing to do, he brought us back to Hamadan that evening and we booked into the hotel, after which we went shopping. We found that we could get khaki trousers and jackets quite cheaply. The engineer came with us and showed us how to barter and advised us never to pay what we were asked. There was a bazaar in downtown Hamadan with all kinds of trinkets, copper, pewter and brass plates, cups, candlesticks etc., some of which were being manufactured actually in the bazaar. We spent much time watching these artisans beating out plates and cups with their hammers.

In another shop we saw a man making a trunk out of discarded beer cans. He could hammer the steel of the beer cans flat and then hammer it around plywood. Other shops had shelves packed with ladies' underwear, men's long johns, belts, hats and gloves. It was indeed a very entertaining trip. Bob and I bought some trousers and shirts, also of khaki, that would be more serviceable than the clothes we had brought from Europe. White shirts and woollen clothes were going to be of little use and would certainly not last long the way we were living. We also got some big boots that came halfway up our calves, as hiking around in the mud of our camp had practically ruined our British shoes. There was nowhere that we could find that we could have cleaning done, but we were informed that we could wash the trousers and shirts that we had bought. The following morning we had Nestlé's coffee and soft fried eggs and rice with Iranian bread for breakfast in the Bou Ali Hotel. The drive back to Avej was interesting as it was daylight. The road was paved for about 5 miles out of Hamadan but after that it was completely rough. We met some heavy trucks which hardly gave us enough room to pass. The engineer drove a Land Rover, which was fairly comfortable as there were cushions on the seats.

Bob and I whiled away the next few days as best we could. He had a radio, which he had bought in Teheran before coming down the road. He could get the BBC in the evenings as long as we remembered the time difference between Iran time and Greenwich Mean Time. England seemed a long way away and the reception was intermittent, coming and going, waxing and waning, but it was nice to hear the BBC's voices even if it did make us a little homesick. There were no telephones and only a bus which passed twice a day, once going south, probably to Hamadan, and once going north to Teheran. Many trucks passed but none stopped. The bus would stop on request and some of the workers who were going to Teheran or even to Avej would flag it down.

Our ambulance finally arrived with a very polite driver who could speak fairly good English. He had an allowance and could buy petrol and have the ambulance serviced as needed without our getting involved in the expenses.

We set up surgery hours from 11.00 a.m. until 1.00 p.m., and 5.00 p.m. until 7.00 p.m. We had some patients; some with cuts and some with bruises; one or two with teeth needing to be extracted; some with eye injuries, or sore throats and quite a lot with back injuries. It took some weeks to realize that the old back injury ploy had arrived in Iran and was no different from what I had seen in Ireland and in England in the past. It was Workmens' Compensation all over again and nobody ever seems to recover from an injured back.

There was a form of certificate for time off work for people who had injuries. They were printed in Farsi but had an English translation and they were good for a week. This alone got us working and on a regular basis. We soon got to recognize the chronic backs and chronic knee or elbow injuries etc. Our ambulance driver acted as interpreter. We gradually began to get civilians coming in and treated them as best we could. Having had experience in dispensaries in Ireland, this was no problem, but it was easier here because the medications came in large winchesters ready-made so I did not have to make any concoctions. We had lots of antibiotics, penicillin, cough mixtures, stomach mixtures, pain pills and aspirins. We found that some of the men coming from the town were bringing their wives as well, and children. We asked Dr Flamank what we should do (via letter, as there was a courier who went every few days to Teheran and we could send mail). The engineer brought our mail up from Hamadan, which was our address.

Dr Flamank replied that we were to continue to look after the civilians as it was going to bring us considerable goodwill, and as we lived out in such a remote area this was going to be useful. This was true because occasionally we got chickens and vegetables brought in by the people who came to get treated (shades of Ireland).

There was a kitchen in the engineers' building, and Bob fancied his cooking ability, so boiled chicken was a novelty. At the beginning we had been having meals in the contractor's building and they were very enjoyable except that they were enormous. I just couldn't stomach the gigantic antipasto and spaghetti dinners which were put up by the Italian contractor. He had all the workers in there at big tables in the ranch house. He could not speak English but there was always somebody there who could interpret. We were certainly never hungry. In the morning the contractor sent over breakfast for us, which we ate in the engineers' office.

After a month Bob was not any better and his headache was persistent; next he developed abdominal pains, which were relieved by antacids. My diagnosis was that he had an ulcer.

We asked the contractor to let us pay for our meals but he was highly insulted, so we decided that we could no longer continue to sponge on him. We just could not make him understand what we really meant but eventually he agreed to send us our dinner over to the engineers' office each day. The meals which were being sent over were nothing like the meals that were being served in his ranch house and consisted mostly of fried vegetables and food that I had never seen before. There was a lot of rice and occasionally spaghetti. By the time we got it it was usually quite cold and we did not have the means by which to heat it up. This didn't help Bob's ulcer at all so I sent him up to Teheran to be seen by Dr Flamank. He had taken all his goods and chattels with him because he obviously had no intention of coming back. During the time I was alone the contractor again had me to eat with him as he obviously had drawn the distinction between the doctor and the nurse.

A few days later a new nurse arrived, a Mr Wallace. He was a six-foot Scotsman with a huge head of hair, untrimmed and untidy. He was quite pleasant and I brought him with me to the contractor's dinner. Unfortunately he put his feet up on the table, which upset the contractor no end. It was back to meals in the engineers' office.

Bob Loughman, we heard, had been X-rayed and examined in Teheran and was found to have a fractured skull as well as a peptic ulcer. He was sent home post-haste. I had one letter from him telling me he felt much better and he was not going to return to Iran.

About this time I wrote to my parents and told them where I was. My mother sent me white shirts, and underwear, socks and everything she thought I would need as I had told her what the climate was like. Incidentally, the climate at this time was cold and we had frequent snow, it being the end of January and beginning of February. The socks and underwear were very welcome. Avej was very high and it was a climb of about 5 miles from the south, and then there was a plateau with a gradual descent again going towards Ghazvin on the way to Teheran.

I had written to Gloria to send me some more underwear and long johns, which I had left in Ireland thinking I was going to a desert climate and it would be like the Sahara. It was desert in that there was no greenery and there was brown soil underneath the snow but it would be another month or six weeks before the snow melted and we could get a proper look at the countryside. Otherwise it was like Siberia.

My son Garvan had made friends with a boy called Joey Ray whose father, an Englishman, had married an Irish woman and they had bought a farm not far from where we lived. Joey's mother used to take him to school and pick up Garvan and Keevsa on the way and drop them off in the evenings again on the way home. Until I left, we had a maid who used to take them to school. We then discharged the maid as I figured that Gloria could look after the house full-time. I wrote to Mrs Ray and told her where I was and what I was doing, and almost by return she wrote to me. She told me that she had called in one evening to see Gloria and give her some company and talk to her. She said she had given her some advice to stay and watch the children, and the way she put it was, 'She was a little sleepy, but she wasn't too bad. I advised her not to drink outside the home as she had been up in P. Mickey's and had had a few drinks.' Mrs Ray, I knew, was not a narrow-minded woman and liked to take a drink herself, so I knew by this that Gloria must have been pretty well stoned.

Next, I got a letter from the local school teacher who told me that she did not live far away and when my children had not come to school she went down after school to find out why. She found the children at home alone eating cornflakes and water. Their mother had not been home the night before and she was still not at home. Apparently, the children had spent the previous evening alone and it transpired that Gloria had slept up in the pub, not being able to get home. This was not the first occasion and things had been going from bad to worse. Mrs Ray had decided not to get further involved. Mrs McCabe, the schoolteacher, called Gloria's sister Marie in Fintona and told her the story. Marie arrived over hotfoot, to find things were in bad shape and Gloria was drunk again.

Marie wrote to me and told me about this and thought the best thing to do would be to take the children to Fintona with Gloria and clear out the house and leave. I wrote back and told her to do it. I had been disappointed that when I had suggested this before I left, to Marie Bradley, she said she couldn't possibly do that. Now that she had to do it, she could!

I had been sending Gloria money, but nevertheless she had sold the refrigerator and various furnishings in the house to people who had apparently taken advantage of her. She probably sold all the furniture. I never found out where it went or what happened to it except for some valuable silver and wedding presents, clocks, etc., which Marie Bradley took home in her car and probably still has.

I wrote to Mr Fawcett, our landlord, and told him that we would be giving up the house and to let me know whatever rent was owing and I would pay it. I heard from him in about two weeks and paid off the rent. I told Marie to clear out anything else in the house and that I would pay her.

While all this was going on I myself was ready for an ulcer, and my worries and anxieties apparently showed when Dr Flamank came down to visit me on his way down the line to check on the hospitals. I told him my situation. He was very sympathetic but he said he would not recommend me going home and as a matter of fact he forbade me to go home. He said if I left I would not get back as Amman & Whitney had my passport and it would be difficult to get my fare paid back, etc., etc. He did me a favour because if I had gone home I would have gone home to disaster.

Marie Bradley had now taken over the situation, and in spite of her refusing to help me out when I was leaving, she now was saddled with my family and they were safe. I continued to send home payments, but instead of sending them to Gloria I sent them to Marie with instructions to give Gloria spending money only.

I found that I could catch a bus to Teheran on a Thursday and be back early on Saturday, as Friday was the Moslem sabbath. I paid a visit to Amman & Whitney's office and saw Betty. She was very helpful and invited me over to her apartment with some of the other doctors who were in town and we had a party. I was the closest field hospital to Teheran, so it was easy for me to get up and back down to Avej at weekends. When a new doctor came, I happened to be in Teheran and met him in the office. We had another party over in Betty's apartment and he turned out to be a wonderful tenor singer. There was a hamburger restaurant near the office, called the Rainbow Room, and Betty and I had eaten there before, so we brought Dr Turner down and had some beer and hamburgers. After that we went to a *pension*, had some more drinks and took Dr Turner back to his hotel. Betty invited me to stay in her apartment as she had an extra room with a folding cot. It was very comfortable and she had a fridge full of food and beer, vodka, scotch and everything that was necessary to make a party. There was a wonderful rooftop patio attached to Betty's apartment and it was very pleasant to sit out there as it was cool but not too cold.

When I returned to Avej I had a bottle of vodka which, by the way things were going in Ireland, I needed. From then on Betty kept me and my nurse supplied with vodka, gin, biscuits and various foods that she was able to get from the PX, to which she had access through Amman & Whitney, who had the privilege through the Corps of Engineers. Mr Wallace, the Scotsman, complained about the food and was generally discontented with his situation, so he was transferred elsewhere and Dr Flamank sent down a Mr Harris, a male nurse, who had recently arrived. My association with him was a great improvement. He was very knowledgeable and adaptable and efficient. He had apparently been a head nurse and he was well acquainted with the operation of hospital emergency rooms and surgery.

We had an interesting experience one night. We heard a knock on the door and outside there was an Iranian gentleman, well dressed, looking like a businessman. He had apparently gone to the main camp office and to the contractor's house and asked if there was a doctor available. One of his friends had injured his arm while changing a wheel on the way down from Teheran when they had a flat tyre. We invited him in and, as it was a cold night, we invited them all in. There were four of them. The man's arm was checked and found to be okay, not broken, but we gave him some aspirin and pain medication to carry him through as they were on their way to the Gulf and they had a long trip ahead of them. That night they were going to stay in Hamadan.

They had food in hampers and salads in bowls, and I don't know how it all fitted in the car with the four of them. Anyway, they brought it in and shared it with us. We all got so friendly I asked them if they took a drink, and they did. We produced a bottle of vodka and shot glasses, because vodka was drunk neat in those days in Iran. I filled their glasses and Clive's and mine and we sat down to have a sip. Next thing I knew they had knocked it back in one go, Russian style. So there I was with four empty glasses and Clive Harris and I still with our glasses full. All I could do was fill their glasses again and we drank a little more, and next thing they all tipped back. My vodka bottle was getting short shrift so not to be left out, we decided to knock ours back too. The bottle was soon gone and I didn't produce anything else, knowing that that was going to happen. We told them we had no more. Having got loosened up, they went out to their car and came in with another bottle, which we all enjoyed, and ate all their food, biscuits, cheese and salads. I don't know how they got to Hamadan but they were certainly able to drink and didn't seem any the worse.

The following day I told one of the engineers, an Armenian, a very agreeable man with whom we had become friendly, and he had a few helpers with him. He told us where there was the nearest thing they could get to a pub. We hadn't known about this so we all got into the ambulance, went up and got into this pub. It was just a bare room with seats around the walls. No tables. The engineer told them what we needed and they came out with a bottle of arak (the Iranian vodka). We all had a drink and we bought a bottle, and they also had Iranian beer, Shams. We loaded up and got back to the camp. We nearly ended up drinking as much vodka as the night before, but the engineer knew not to knock it back and we all sipped, unlike our previous night's visitors. The following morning, however, the difference between the arak and the vodka we were getting from Teheran became apparent. Harris and I had severe headaches. The native-made vodka was a bit like poteen, the illicit whiskey made in Ireland. The effects were much the same. If you drank water the following day, you got sozzled again. The beer was heavy and it was in large bottles, at least a pint, probably a litre. They didn't measure pints in Iran.

It was about two or three weeks after the visit by the strangers in the car that they arrived again, a bit earlier in the evening. This time they had come prepared for a party. They had a big bowl of salad on ice, a case of vodka and all kinds of delicacies and Iranian food, which they carried into the engineers' office. They laid it on the table and we all sat around and had a really great party. Between the four of them, Clive and me, I think we finished two bottles of vodka, and when the party was over they left us two bottles with apologies for having drunk us out the first time. They went on their way. I don't know whether they were going to Teheran or Hamadan, but we never saw them again.

On another occasion we had a visit by a doctor from Morrison Knudsen Organization, who had a project going about halfway between Hamadan and Avej. I am not sure what they were building – it was either a factory or an airfield – but it was about 2 miles off the road and could not be seen. As long as we knew where to turn off the main road and go over a hill, this enormous camp was there, surrounded by a high fence and a guard at the gate to whom we had to give our identification and justify our visit. Our visit was a return visit to the English doctor who was in charge of the medical unit at the camp. When he had visited us in Avej we had had some drinks. Other than that, our hospitality was limited as we had not much access to food. He invited us down to his unit and told us how to get there. We arrived one evening and went into a big mess, which was more like an army mess than anything else. There was a buffet, from which we helped ourselves. All he had to do was to say we were his guests, so Clive and I and he had a very good meal. At least, better than anything we were getting in Avej.

We then went to his quarters, where he had a very comfortable apartment, record player, radios etc. He played records, all the up-to-date music of the time, and he had lots of liquor. We had whisky, American beer and bourbon and it was a very enjoyable evening. We left after midnight and it was such a clear, starry night that it was easy to drive back. We were told that any time we went to Hamadan to drop in, not to pass. Not being able to return the compliment, we visited very rarely.

Dr Turner, the singer, had arrived and Dr Flamank decided that he would put him in charge of a hospital on the road between Hamadan and Khorramabad. Another clinic had been established in Hamadan in which he put a Dr French in charge. Whenever we now went to visit Hamadan we had somewhere else to call, other than the Bou Ali Hotel and another hotel down the street in which there was a nightly cabaret.

The Bou Ali was a beautiful hotel and it seemed to me at the time to be enormous. The main lobby was surrounded by balconies, which gave access to the rooms. When one went into a hotel room, from the windows there was a marvellous view of mountains and surrounding hills in the distance. The hotel was three-storey and it extended probably over a block, with nice gardens designed in an Iranian architectural style.

Hamadan was built like a cartwheel, with streets going out from the centre to the periphery. Interconnecting the spokes of the cartwheel would be other streets, with streets between them. They were wide streets and the shopping area was toward the centre of the town, where the bazaar was also situated. Not far from the hotel was the clinic, and almost next door to the clinic was a guest house run by a Swiss company. We met an architect from that company in the Bou Ali Hotel bar and became friendly with him, but shortly after that he was transferred. The next time I met him was in the Canary Islands on my way back from Africa to London.

About March or April the snow began to melt and some leaves appeared on the trees in a little wood beside the camp. It was a relief to get away from the monotony of the snow. On my walks in the surrounding countryside I discovered about three villages. The houses were mostly made of mud, with few windows and quite forbidding. The streets between them were extremely narrow, and were it not for the fact that the villages were so small, one could get lost. Each village was surrounded by a wall. It was said that each village belonged to a land owner, who owned not only the village but the villagers as well.

In the spring and summer the villagers planted crops around the outside of the village in fields, which they tilled. They were paid by getting a portion of the crop in the form of food. It was said that someone who didn't work was put outside the walls in the winter in the snow and the wolves came and ate them. We could not believe that happened in our day and age but, noting how well disciplined the villagers were, it might indeed have been a possibility.

There was a village near the camp called Garmac and in June the landlord gave a party in the little wood beside the camp. Lights had been hung from the trees and a barbeque was going. We were all invited. Apparently it was thrown for the contractor and employees of the camp. We had kabobs, which were excellently done but the meat was a bit tough. I presumed it was lamb, probably mutton, and some chicken. There was wine and, of course, a big urn of tea, which was the drink that the Iranians usually had, laced with a lot of sugar. It was served in small cups, or glasses, and usually too hot to hold if it was filled to the top. In each glass or cup at least three lumps of sugar were dropped before it was given to you. The party was a quiet affair because it was outdoors and there was not much room for hilarity. After it was over we went to the workers' quarters attached to the ranch house. I now realized that the food we were getting was the food for the labourers, who lived in very, very primitive circumstances. However, they were all a merry bunch and there were quite a number of Armenians and some Russians. One of them had an accordion. This was the first time I had seen the Armenians dancing. They danced Russian dances with their arms folded, dancing from a squatting position. It was very enjoyable. They sang songs in their native languages and the Russians joined in and sang Russian songs to the accompaniment of the piano accordion.

There were chessboards there and one of the Russians asked me if I played chess. I thought I did and said so. He beat me in five moves. I played him again, and he beat me in about seven. I didn't want to play him again and I don't think he was interested in playing me again either. That put me off chess for life. I have never played much since.

We got friendly with the people at the party and that included some of the natives from the villages. One day I got an emergency call to go and see a woman patient in Garmac village. I took what I thought I would need in a medical bag. I took thermometers, blood pressure apparatus etc., and my interpreter, who was currently a young man from Avej who could speak a little English. I did not know what I was letting myself in for or what to expect, but we brought the ambulance as far as we could get on the road and walked the rest of the way. The husband brought us through a lot of back alleys and we eventually got to the house. It looked nothing from the outside but inside it seemed very comfortable indeed. There were carpets on the floor, around the walls, on the table – everywhere you could see was carpeted. Apparently, your wealth is in carpets. You don't put your money in a bank you put it in carpets.

Anyway, I had a look at this lady in a back room. Her bed was on the floor, not raised. It was very embarrassing and difficult because the lady was fully clothed and her husband didn't want her undressed in front of a stranger. I told him to get some of the women in, and they allowed me to slide a stethoscope under her clothes and listen to her heart and lungs. I found nothing gross there but her abdomen was definitely tender. She looked about 40 years of age but she was probably about 30. Iranian women do not wear well, probably as the result of doing all the work around the house and getting very little exercise outside and living virtually as slaves.

My differential diagnosis was appendicitis or a tubal pregnancy or diverticulitis or renal calculus, because I had to examine her through her clothes and it seemed all her pain was in her right side. She was running a temperature of about 101° so I told her husband that she was seriously ill and that she should be in hospital.

In the town of Avej there was an Iranian doctor, whom I never met, but he had a name-plate facing to the street and the house was surrounded by a high wall. I was told that there was some form of clinic there where the doctor saw patients every so often. I recommended that they either bring her to him or to Hamadan. Having had experience of the hospital in Hamadan, I thought the doctor in Avej might be the best bet.

I left and they were thankful. I gathered from the interpreter a few days later that they had taken her to Teheran, and it had been arranged by the landlord of the town. That might have been because of my suggestion that they not bring her to Hamadan because I was not impressed with the way the hospital was run.

The lady survived and got home again; apparently it was an appendicitis. Her husband, in his gratitude, and probably the woman herself also, sent us Iranian bread and a form of pie. What was in the pie I don't know but it tasted great, especially with a shot of vodka. Clive was a bit cagey about eating it but I did well on it with no ill effects. A Greek engineer who visited occasionally and sometimes stayed over was there and he helped me finish it. He was in his fifties and was excellent company. He spoke good English and it was a great break from having to speak only to poor Clive and the interpreter, and of course the ambulance driver, who did some of the interpreting.

I became very friendly with the driver as time went on and he introduced me to his cousin, the son of the chief landlord of the town of Avej. This young man's name was Parvis and he took a great liking to me. Although his English was poor, we were able to communicate fairly well, and he invited me to his home for an evening meal. We sat on the floor. He showed me how to sit cross-legged, which was very uncomfortable, but I am sure if I had been younger I could have done it easier and if I had persevered I would have got used to it.

All the men sat around the table, which was almost on the floor, and the women, including his very attractive sister, brought the food. As soon as the food was put down with a glass of tea they left, and the men all sat around and talked and smoked. When the next course was due, someone clicked his fingers and there was a woman apparently standing outside the door. She sent a message to the kitchen to clear the table and bring the next course. I thought I'd never get finished. Courses kept coming and I learned the secret was not to eat all of anything, no matter how hungry one was, because there was plenty more to come; all different, and Iranian food is delicious. Mixtures of vegetables, kabobs, rice, were followed by more salads, fruit and vegetables that I never saw before or since. Attached to the house was a very large garden with paths through it and it looked semi-wild. There were fruit trees, apples, plums, damsons etc., and past that there was a little stream which was running down a hill to the bottom of the valley. It must have been 6 acres and was huge.

Next door to the house was a swimming pool, not really a swimming pool but baths, which the ambulance driver invited me to come and swim in. However, that had to be scratched as it wasn't considered appropriate to let a non-Moslem like me, a Christian or whatever they thought I was, into the same water as the sacred Moslems. It was a religious pool and it looked very attractive. It was not deep but there were seats where one could sit in the water, and the water was heated. However, Clive and I had to settle for our shower in the engineers' building.

As Parvis also had a *chai-khana*, combined with a shop, it was an excuse for us to get away from the camp and go up to Avej. We now had somewhere to go and we could sit in there and have a glass of tea and watch the natives coming and going. There were a lot of cars and trucks going up and down the road and they all stopped and the drivers came in for tea and smoked cigarettes. In the *chai-khana* we could buy nuts, candies and little Iranian cakes and eat a meal. Parvis was usually there and he would come out and talk to us about life outside Iran. He had never been any further than Teheran. I think he was about 24. He began to teach me to speak Farsi and how to read Farsi, but it never really got far.

One day he asked me if I would like to ride a horse. I said, 'Yes, but I have not ridden for fifteen years.' He said he would bring his horse down to the camp and we would go riding. The following day he arrived with two horses and his sister riding a third. We went riding over the hills and it was very pleasant indeed. The horse was fairly docile, but with a little encouragement it would gallop. I was glad I had some experience otherwise I would have come off, but I had an English saddle and it was quite easy to ride. Parvis was like a cowboy, he would gallop around and jump over ditches, hedges or stone walls and he was an expert. His sister was also a good horsewoman.

When the weather improved it was quite hot in Garmac. We would sit outside the engineers' building, which had a little balcony where we could put our chairs facing the sun. Our hospital was now being built and it consisted of a big main clinic, which I suppose could have been called an emergency room, surrounded by about five small rooms, two of which we made into bedrooms and one which was made into a kitchen with an oil-burning stove. We had electric lights as there was a plant, run on diesel, to supply electricity for the camp. There were five patient beds in the main clinic.

We were certainly glad to get out of the engineers' building in June, and we moved all the medical equipment over as we had lots of help. The hospital had been designed by Dr Flamank and it was very well done.

Dr Flamank deserved a lot of credit. He was an extremely good administrator. He was dealing with a lot of difficult people. The nurses and doctors had never been in these primitive circumstances before, although I had had a lot of experience in working in what would be considered primitive conditions, even in those days. I think it might have been my experience in dispensing medication and working in a rural area, as I had described it to Dr Flamank in Dublin, that had prompted him to engage me on the spot in the Gresham Hotel.

The clinics which Dr Flamank had set up were all excellent and where he got the experience or the knowledge as to how to do it I did not ask him. I am sorry I did not. He had a wide knowledge of medicine and surgery and obviously was a good diagnostician because any time I described to him problems which I had encountered, he always came up with a very good differential diagnosis and treatment.

Having been with the National Health Service in Northern Ireland, where getting a patient into hospital was very difficult, often impossible, I had to arrive at my own diagnoses. I did not have access to X-rays or laboratory tests or diagnostic procedures which nowadays would be considered absolutely essential. With the clinic in Iran, I realized that I was much better equipped than I had been in my eight years' practice in Ireland out in the mountains of Tyrone and Fermanagh. Here there were four in-patient beds; there were stains and all the paraphernalia necessary for doing microscopic, histological and bacterial examinations. It was well equipped for surgery and obstetrics, and the medicines supplied were adequate for all but the most unusual medical situations.

Incidental to this, I should mention that in Dr Turner's clinic he had a patient whom he diagnosed as suffering from appendicitis, and the situation was getting much worse as the man was very seriously ill. Dr Turner decided to do an appendectomy, with the nurse giving the anaesthetic. His diagnosis was slightly off. As soon as he opened the abdominal wall, instead of encountering intestines he encountered roundworms. There must have been more than 100, by his description. They were all over the place, they came out of the abdomen, got onto the floor, onto the bed and this would have been unbelievable had I not seen some of them that he had captured and put in a jar in the clinic. The patient had so many worms that they had eventually perforated his intestine.

There was a near riot at the hospital because they accused poor Dr Turner of killing the patient. And although he did not kill him, he got him to a hospital in Hamadan, where he died later. To cool the situation down in that clinic Dr Flamank suggested that I go there and that he move Dr Turner to my hospital. I refused, because I knew that if I went down there my trips to Teheran would be impossible. Unfortunately, this soured the relationship between Dr Flamank and me. I was sorry about that as I had got to like him very much. He was so pleasant and had a wonderful sense of humour and was very kind. The male nurses were constantly complaining about the conditions, the food, the transport etc., and they blamed it all on Dr Flamank. I did my best to explain his situation because he had set up a very good system and programme under very difficult conditions. He was not only dealing with a primitive society but he had to contend with a limited budget and long lines of communication.

For example, going down the line, his first hospital was mine. He got complaints from the engineers that the nurse and I were still in bed at ten o'clock in the morning. Then he got a complaint that we were always in the engineers' office. He wrote me a letter about this and was very apologetic, saying that he would appreciate it if I could be up and out of bed before the engineers arrived and if I wanted to go back to bed after that, it was fine with him. He realized that there really was nothing to do.

The next hospital was in Hamadan where two of the nurses got into a fight and Dr Flamank asked me to go down to straighten out the situation and see what was going on. I arrived down there and I got into a fight with one of the nurses because he was completely unmanageable. I suspected that he was partaking of some of the drugs in the hospital.

Further down the road was Dr Turner's hospital, and he had got into a bad situation with his operation on the man with the worms.

In Khorramabad was the next hospital, and there was a doctor down there who got drunk, became an alcoholic, couldn't be sobered up and had to be sent home.

On the outside periphery he had Dr Butler, who was a very steady, agreeable man and a good doctor. He had, however, got himself a boxer dog, which apparently all the natives were afraid of and they didn't want to go to the clinic when it was there.

Looking back on my experiences in Iran, Dr Flamank was one of the bright spots and he certainly made my stay there very tolerable.

I offered an arrangement to Clive, my nurse, that he could go to Teheran or Hamadan or wherever he wished on alternate weekends and I would go every other weekend. Clive was not interested as he only wanted to save money and have enough to

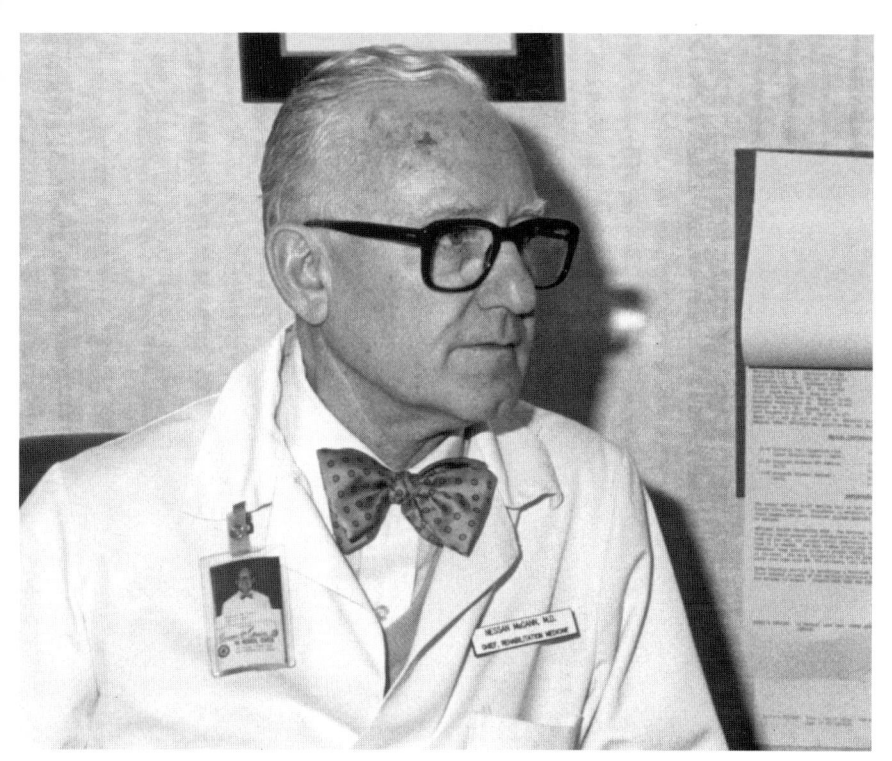

Nessan McCann, M.D.

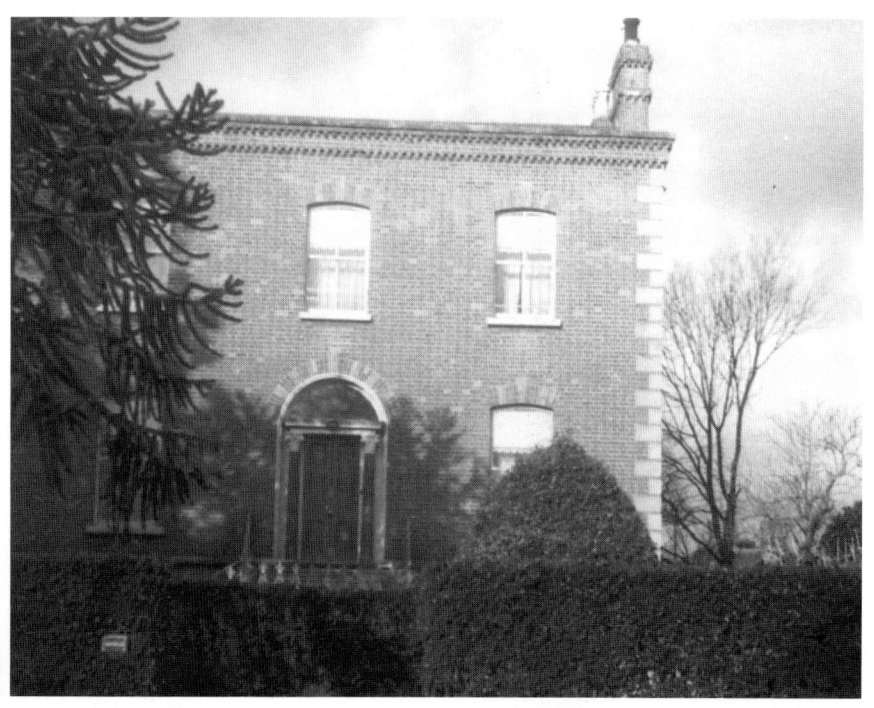

My home in Dublin

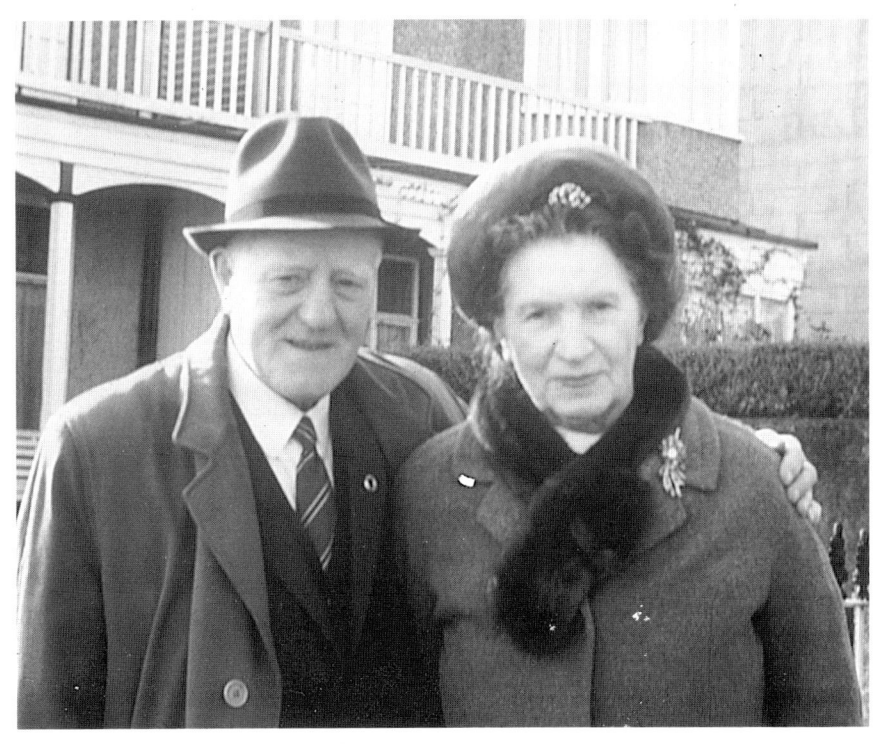

Dr and Mrs Sean McCann (parents)

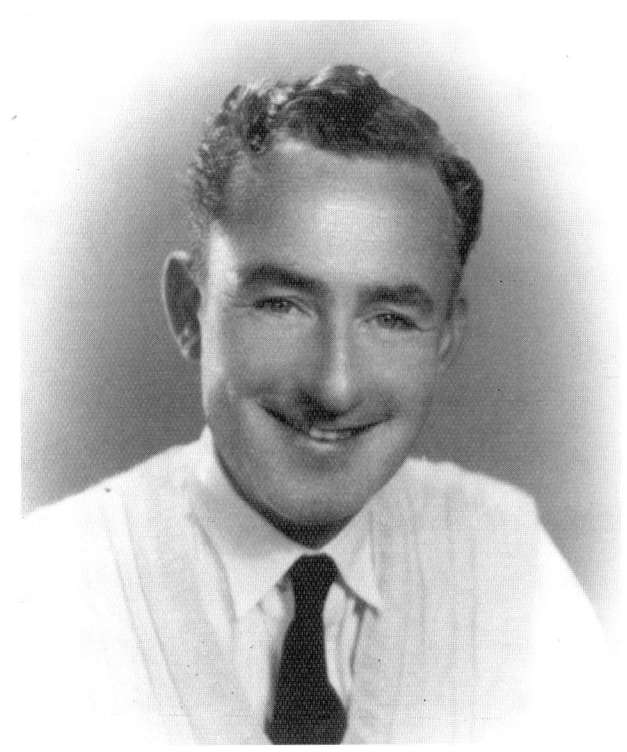

University days

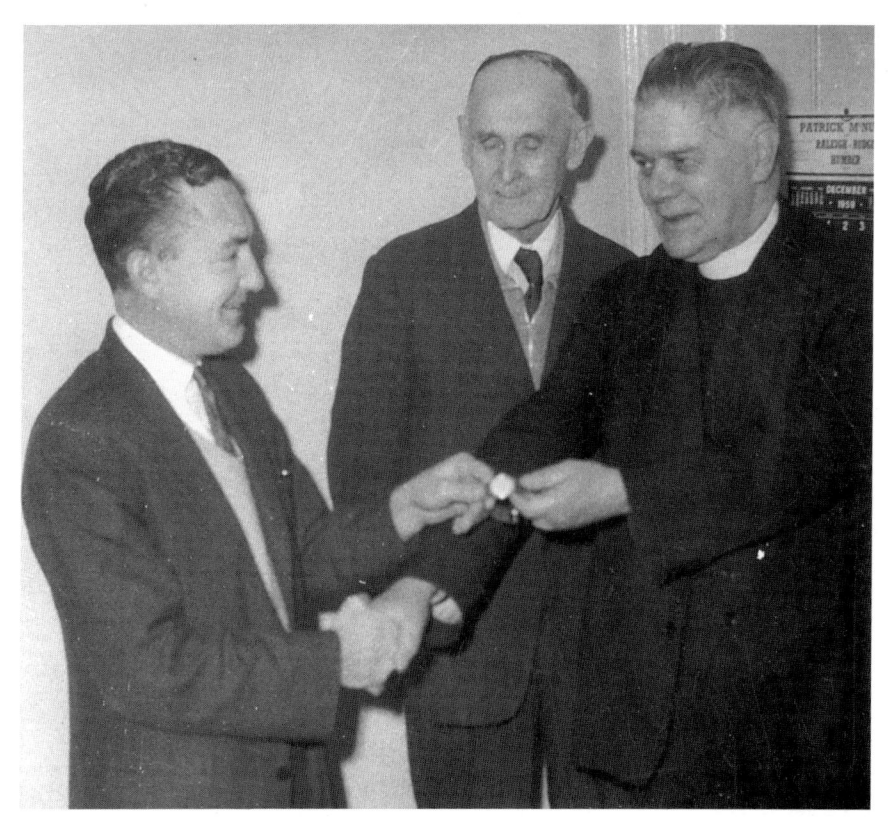

Presentation - Leaving Ireland - 1959

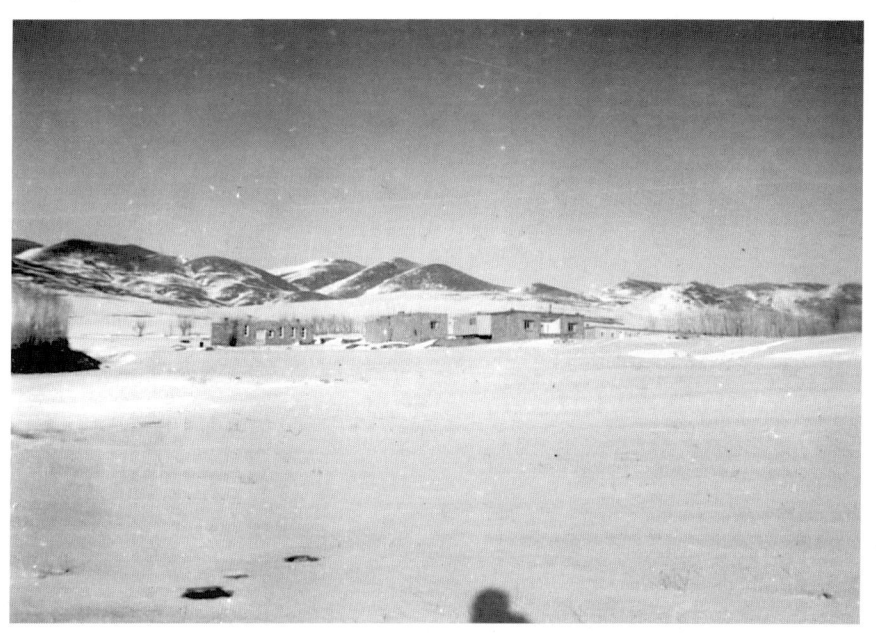

Avej Camp - Iran

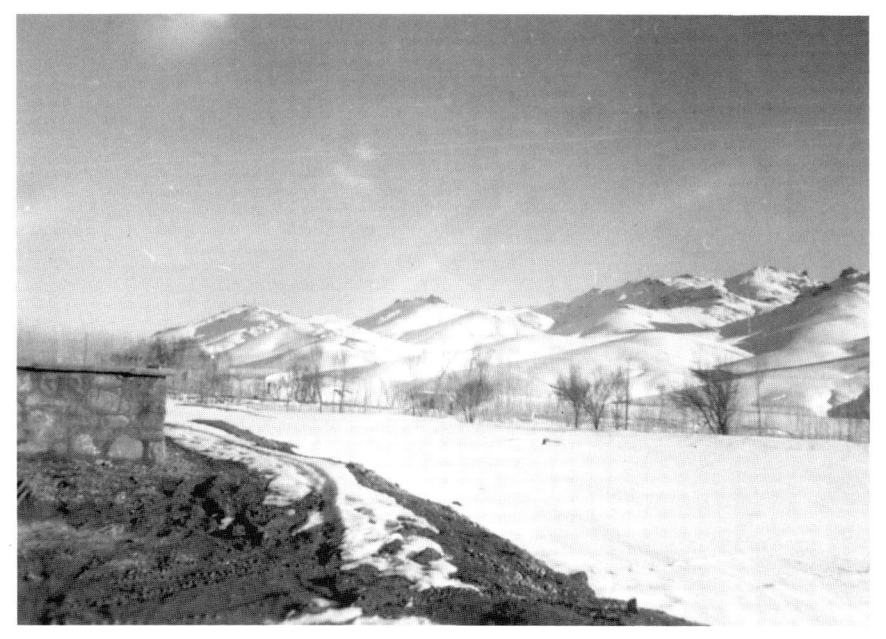

Winter in Avej

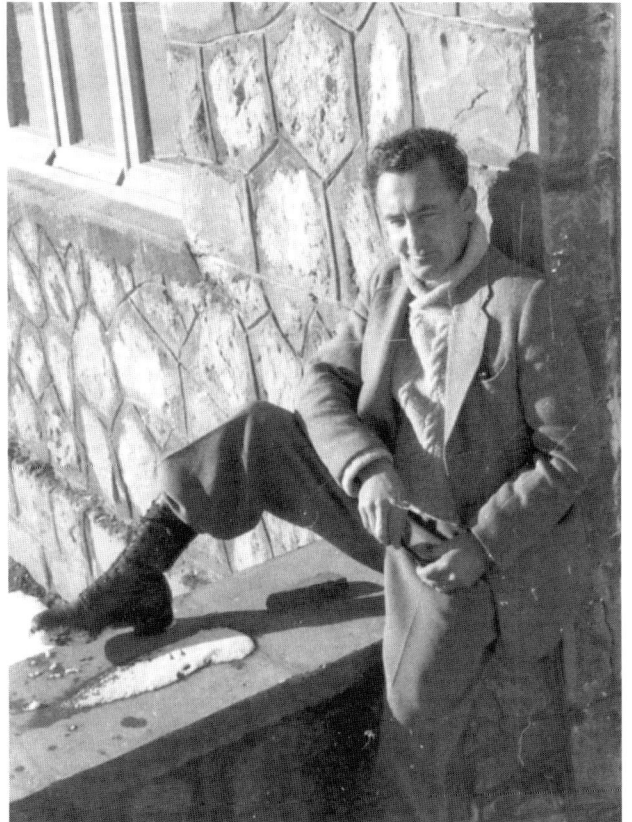

Outside hospital - Avej

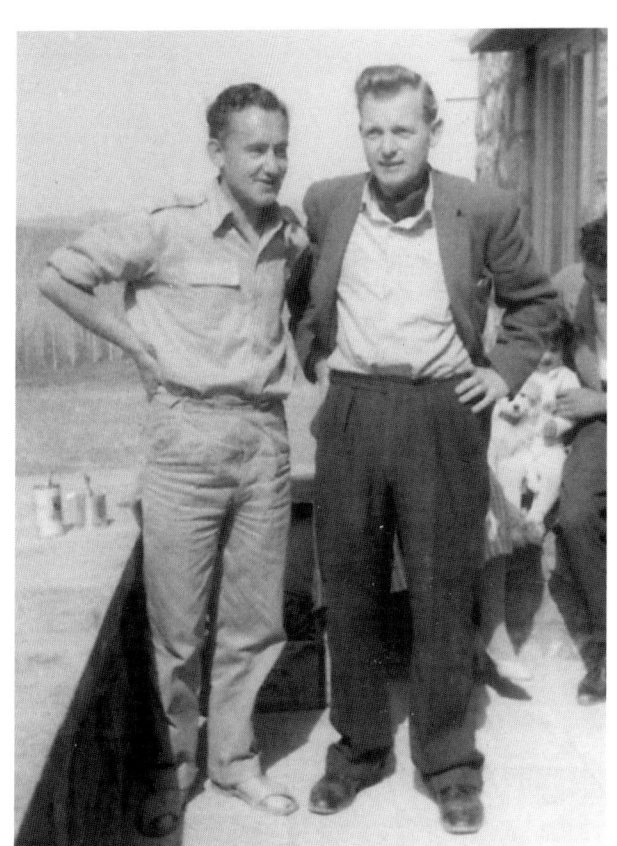

With Morris - male nurse

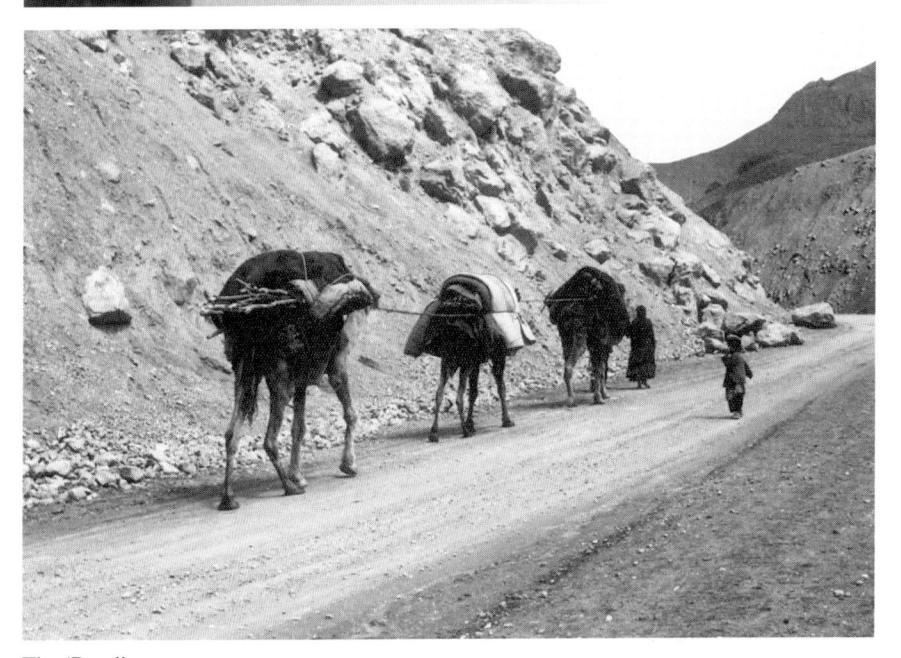

The 'Road'

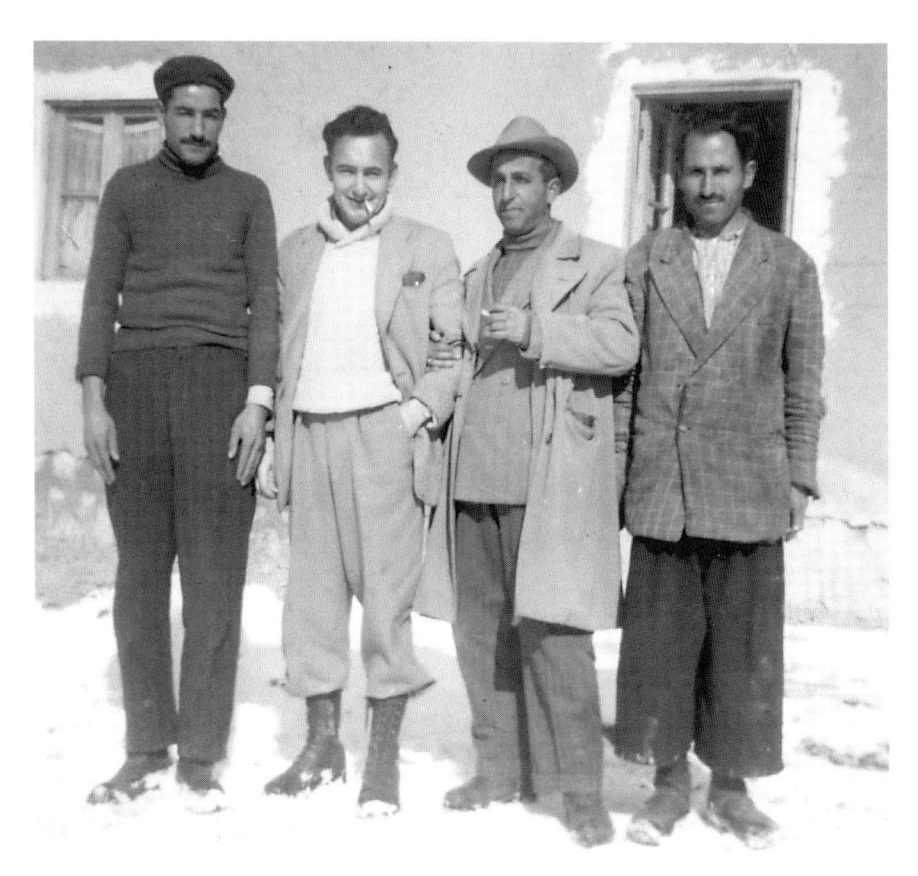

With Avej workers

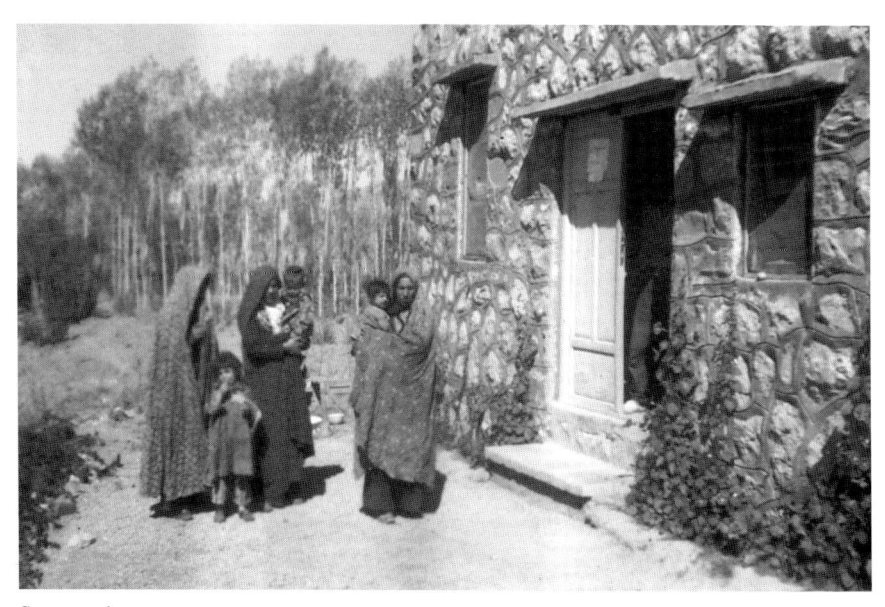

Some patients

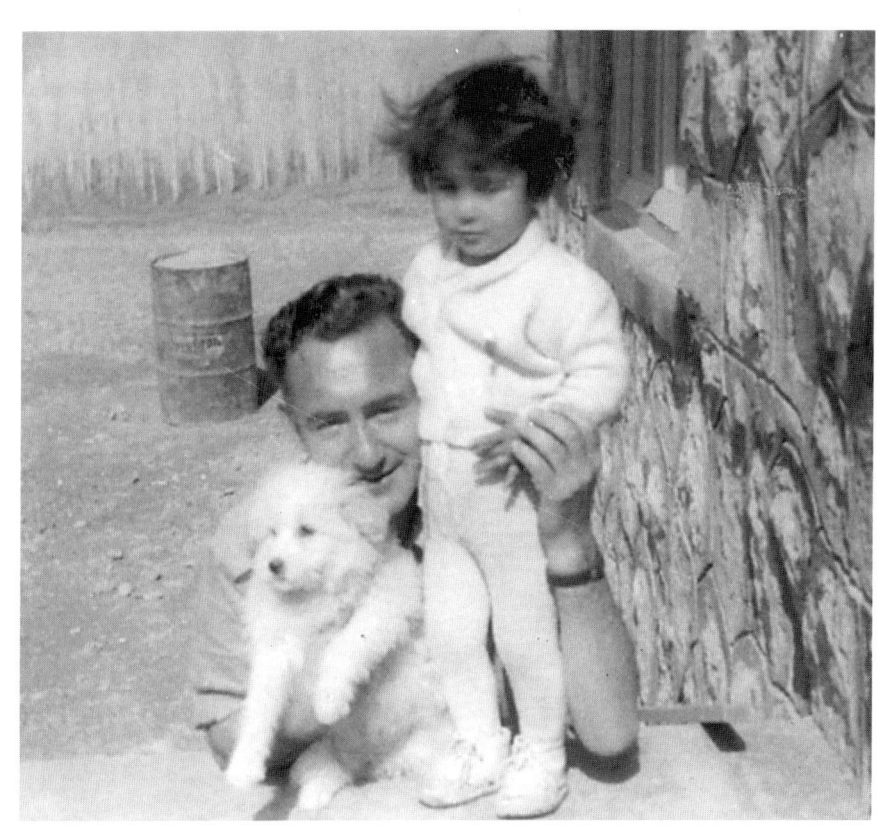

A favourite patient with my dog

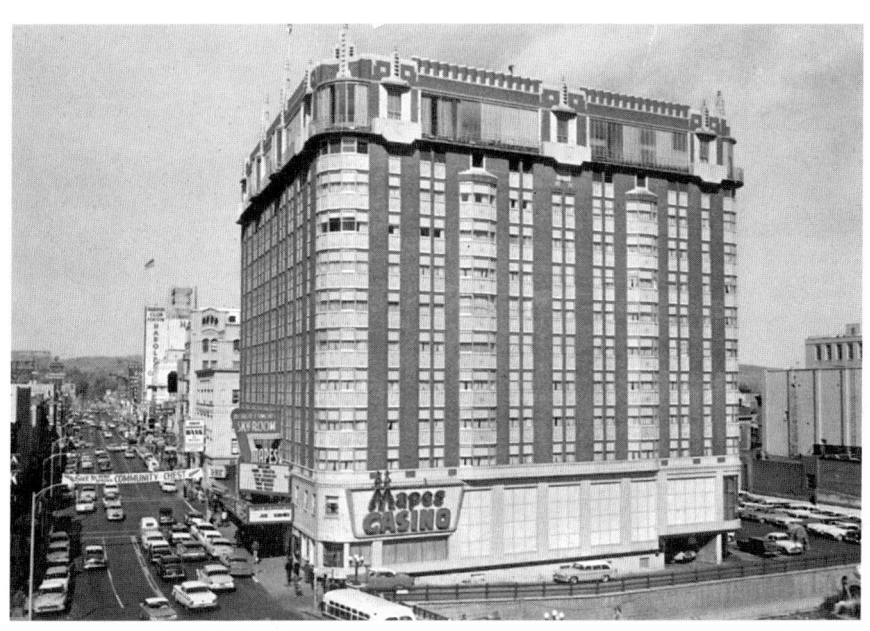

Mapes Hotel - Reno

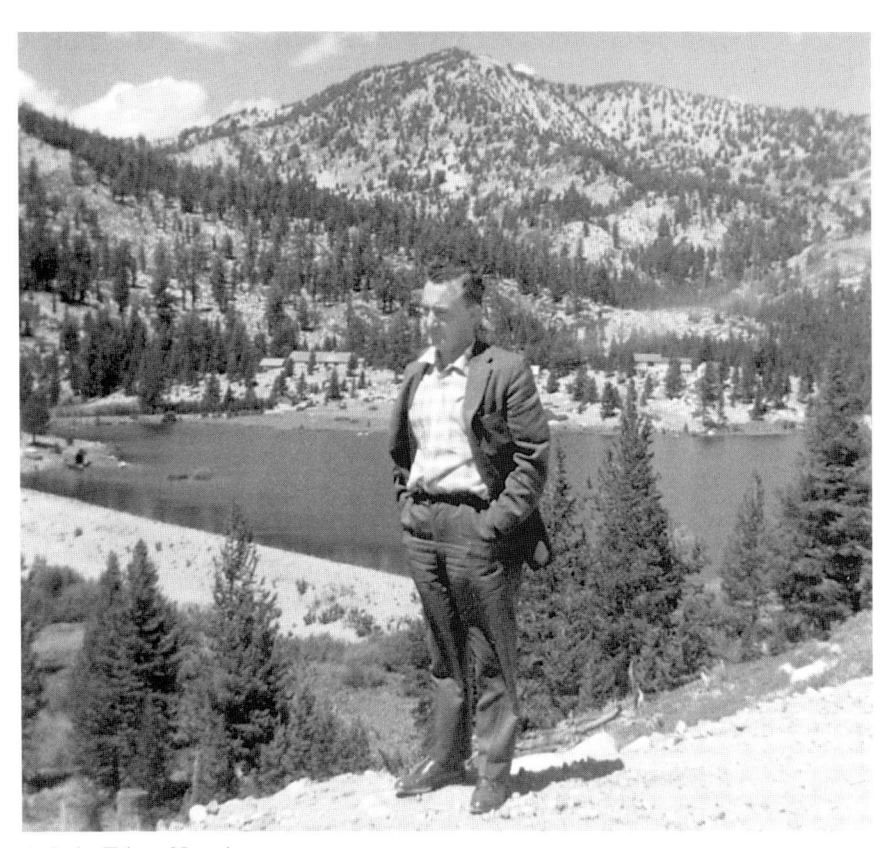

At Lake Tahoe, Nevada

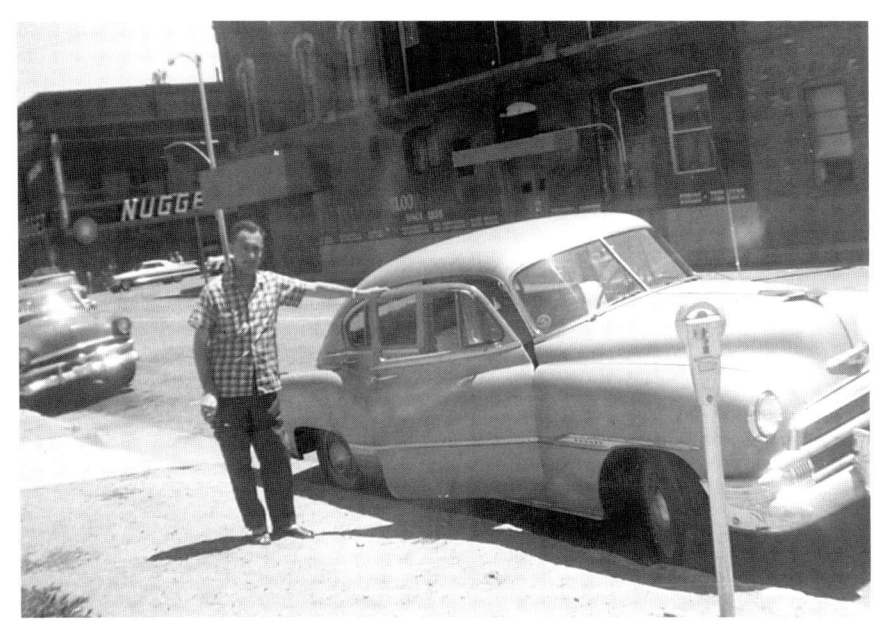

Transport to New York

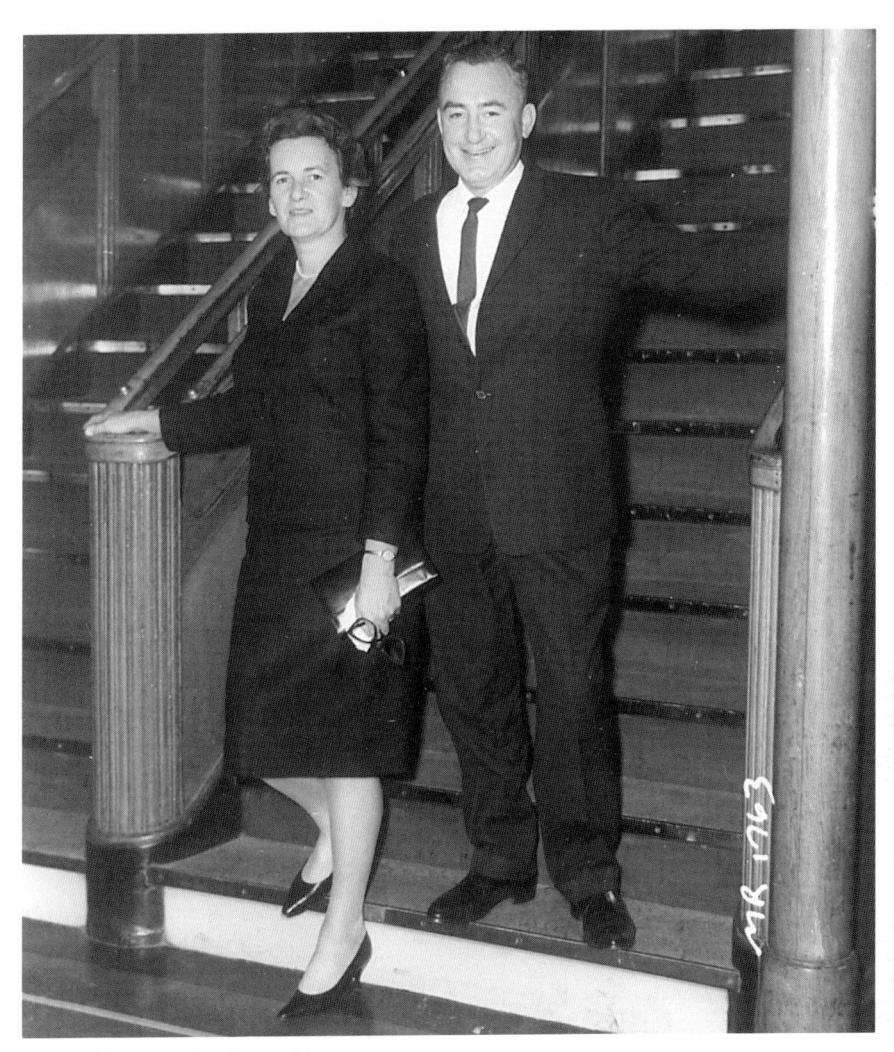

Betty with me on the *Queen Mary*

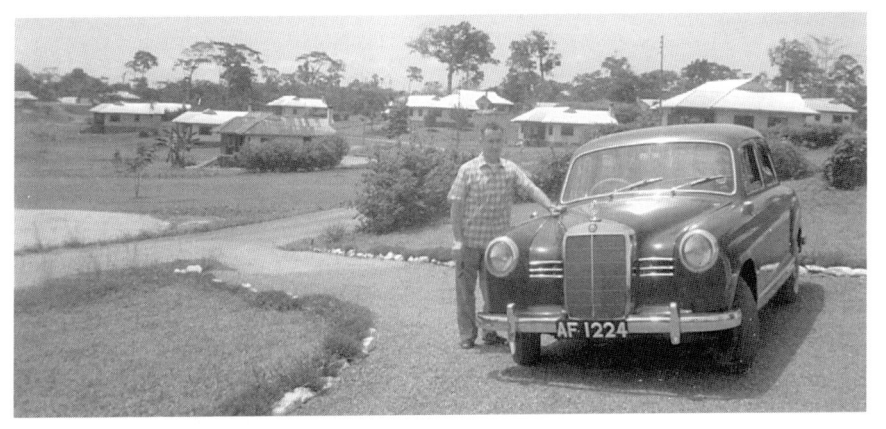

Akwatia compound - diamond mine in Ghana

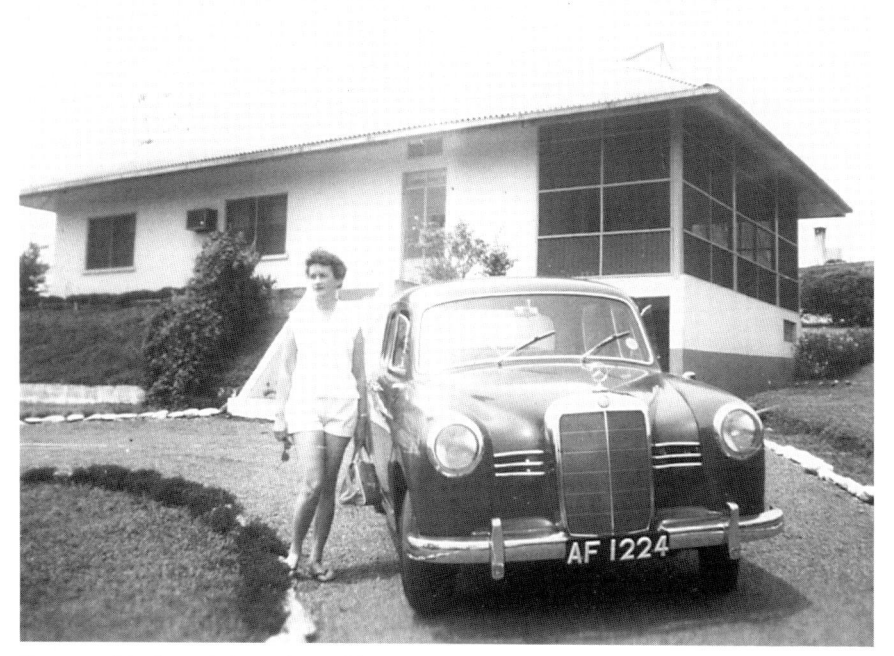

Betty outside doctor's bungalow - Ghana

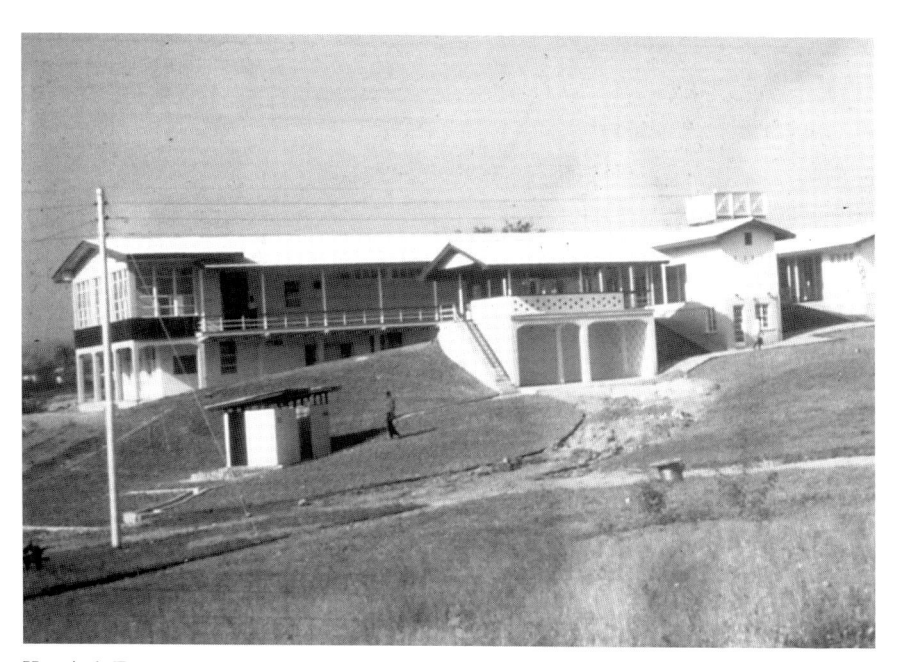

Hospital, Tongo Diamond Mine - Sierra Leone

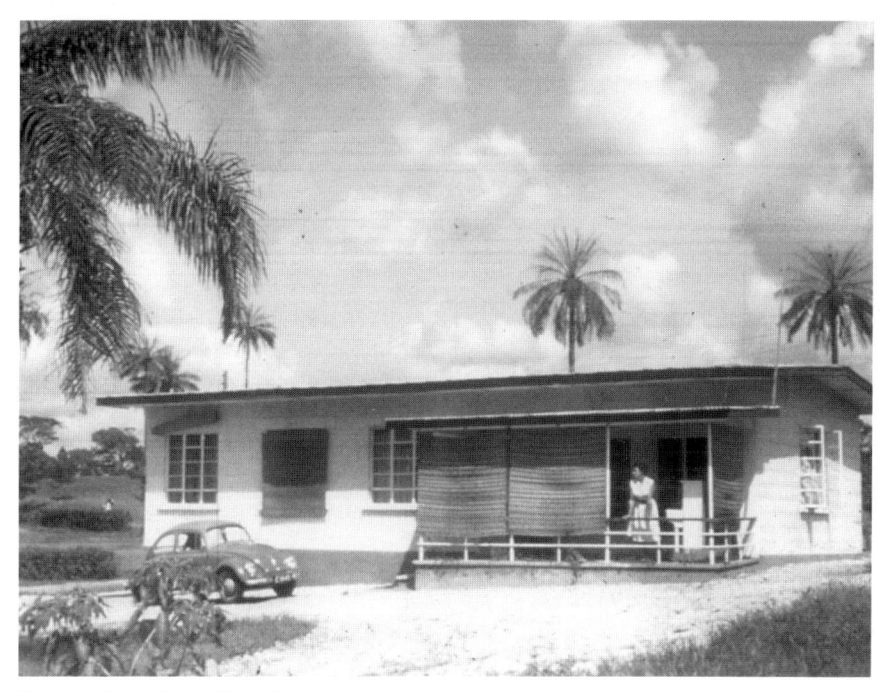

Doctor's bungalow - Sierra Leone

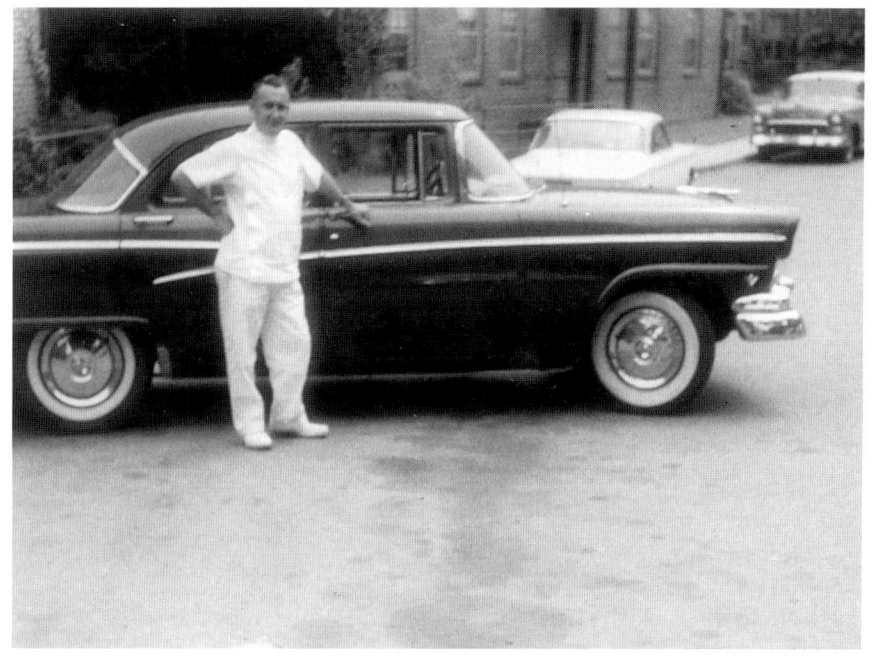

An extern - Norwalk Hospital, Connecticut 1963

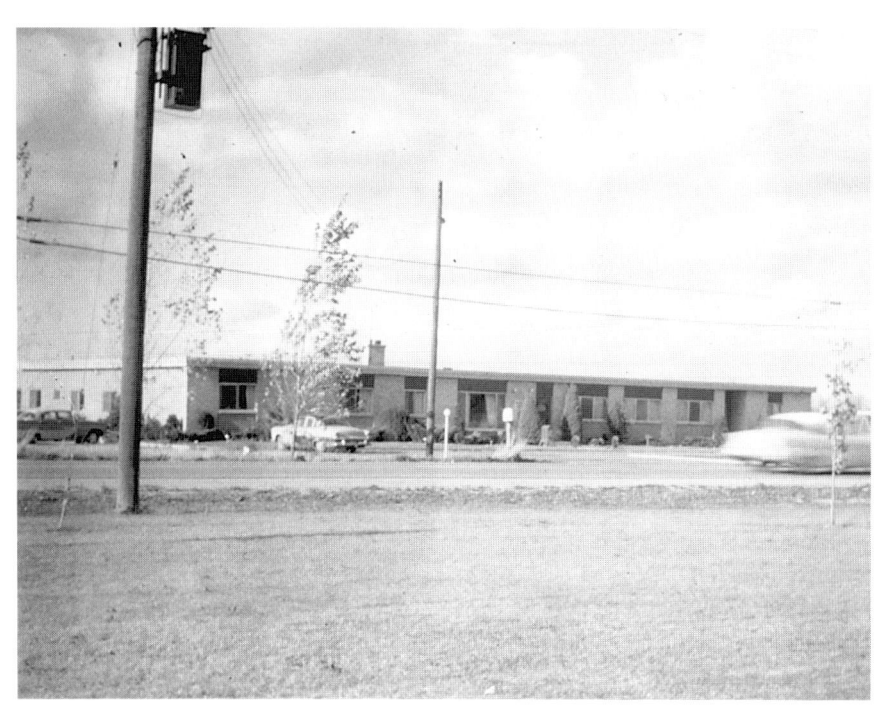

Hospital - Virgil, Canada

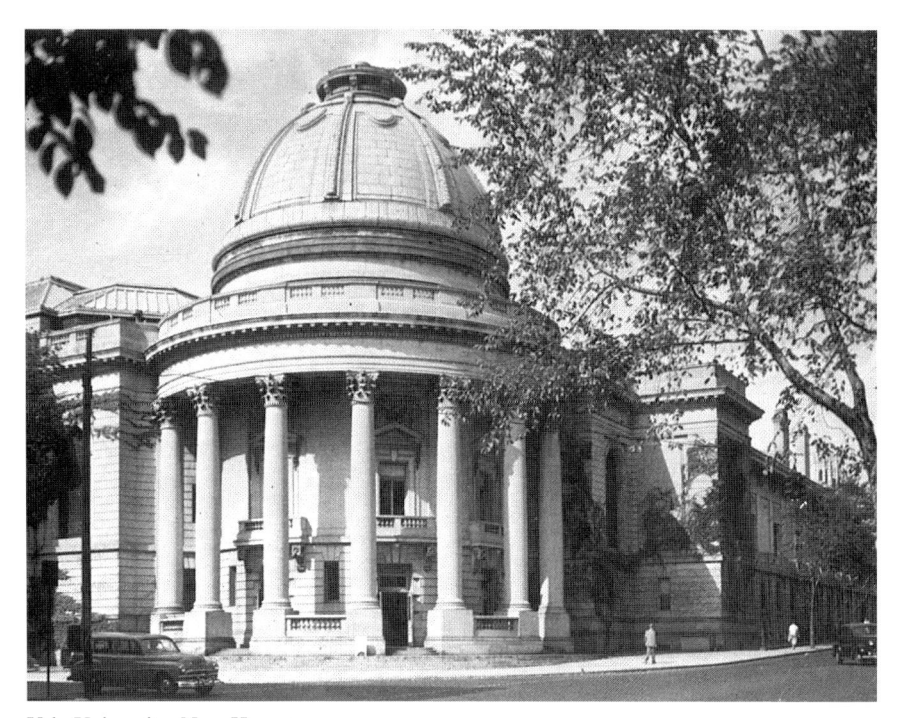

Yale University, New Haven

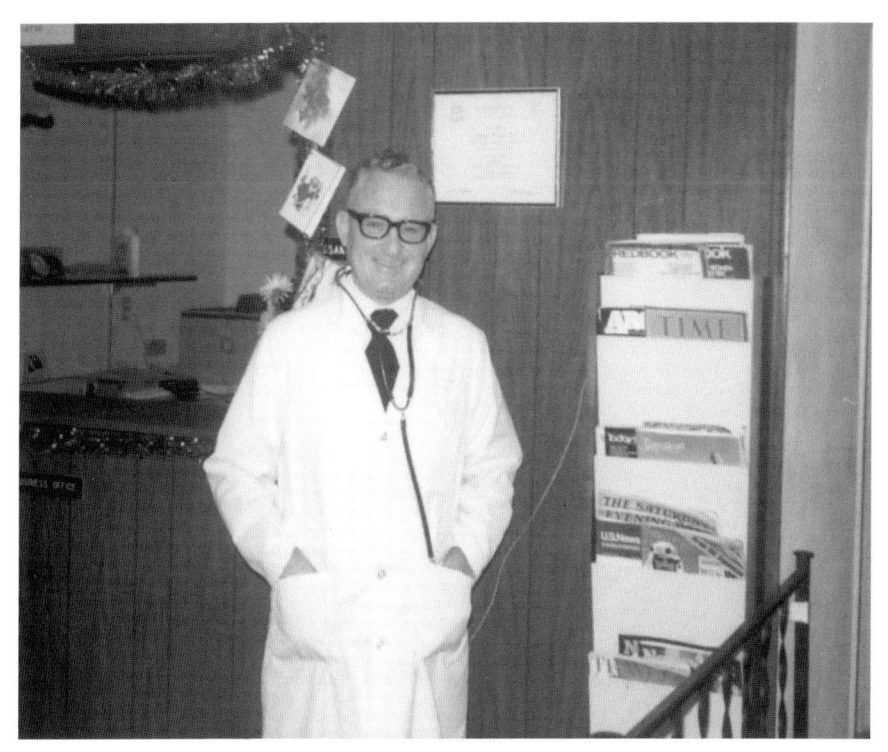

In my office - Holiday, Florida

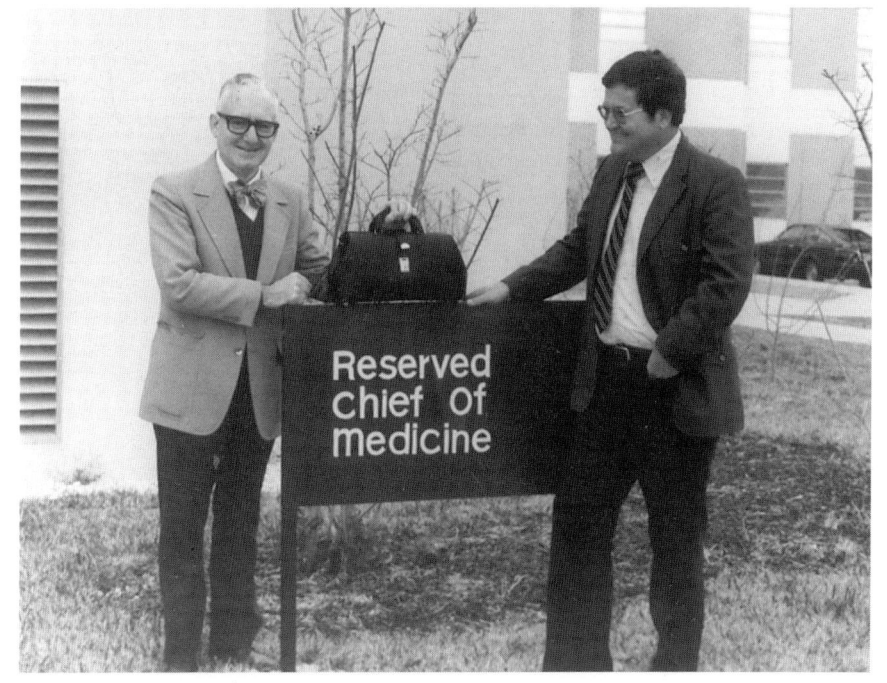

Staking claim - Community Hospital, Florida

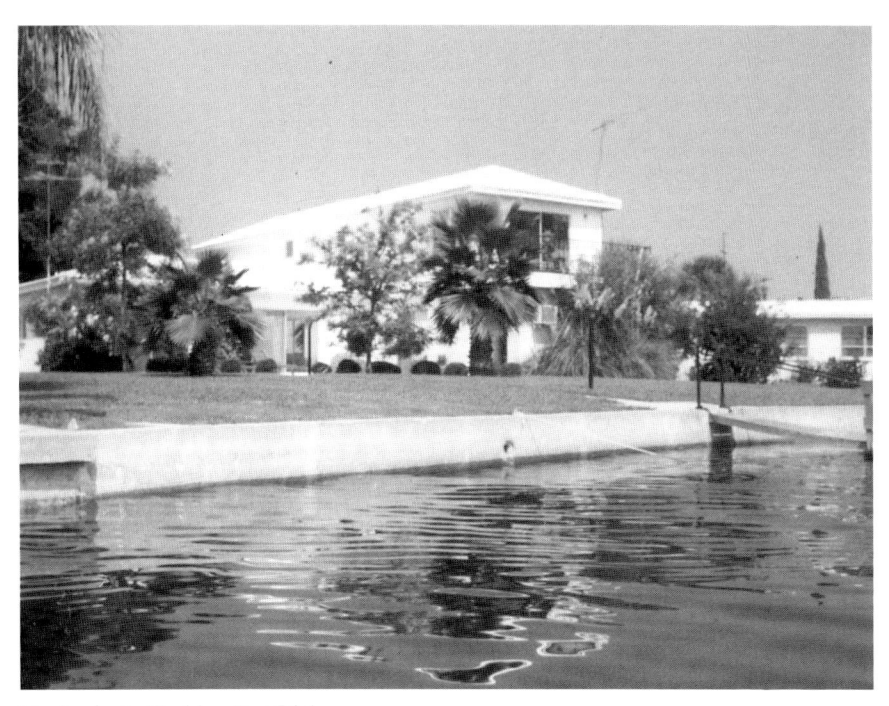

Our house in Florida - Port Richey

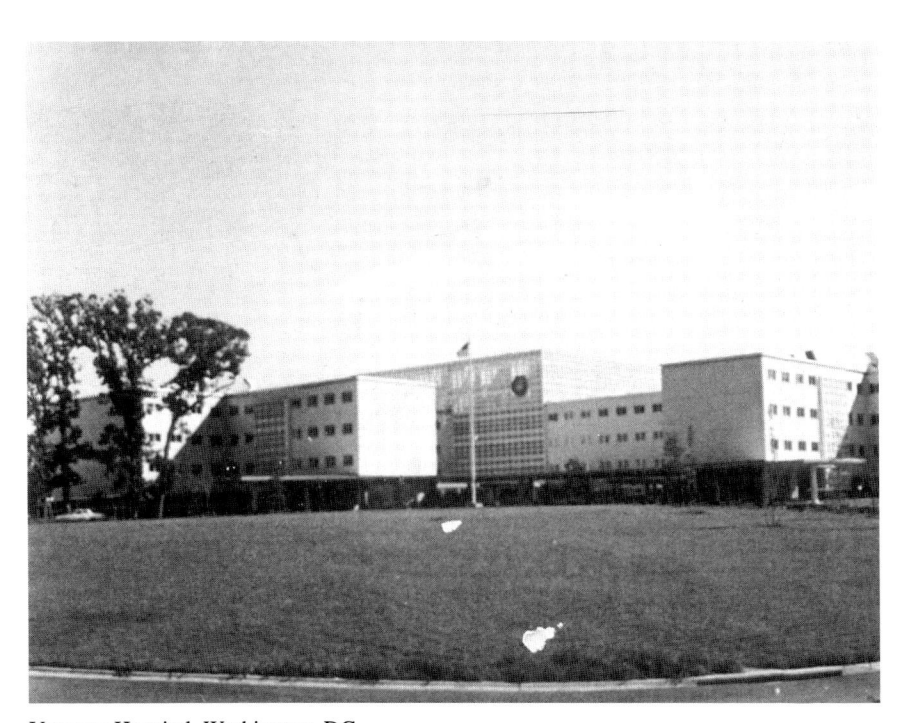

Veterans Hospital, Washington, DC

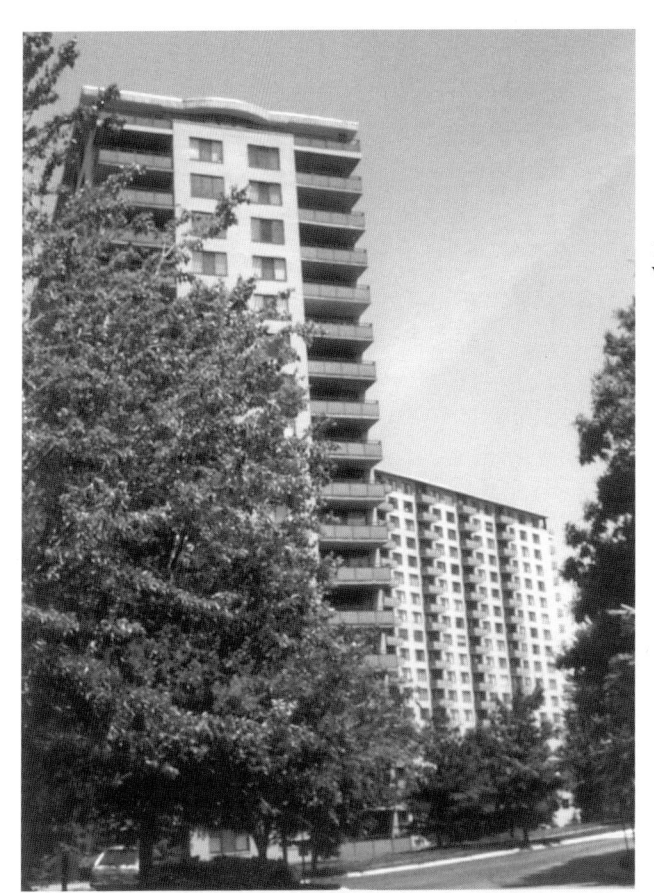

18th floor apartment, Washington

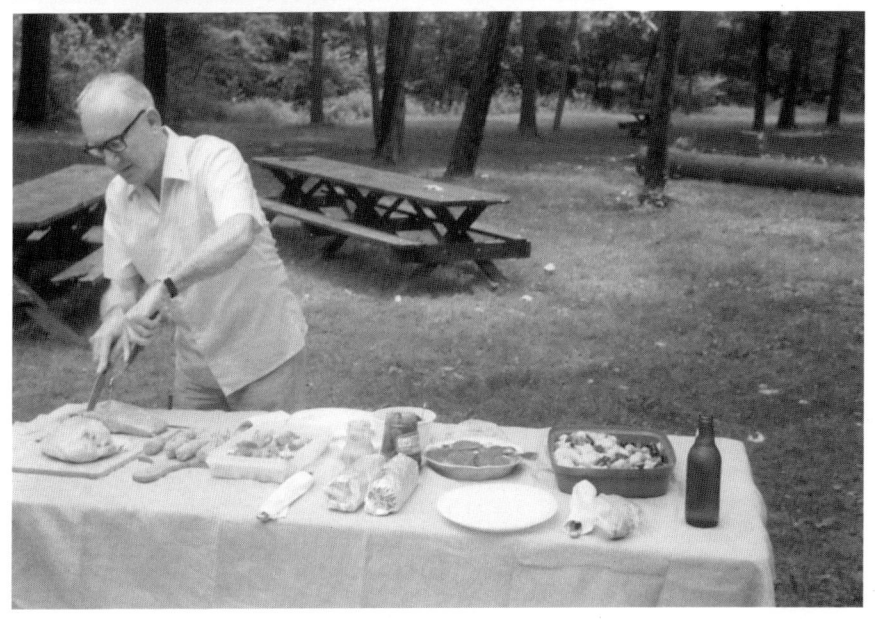

Rock Creek Park picnic - Washington

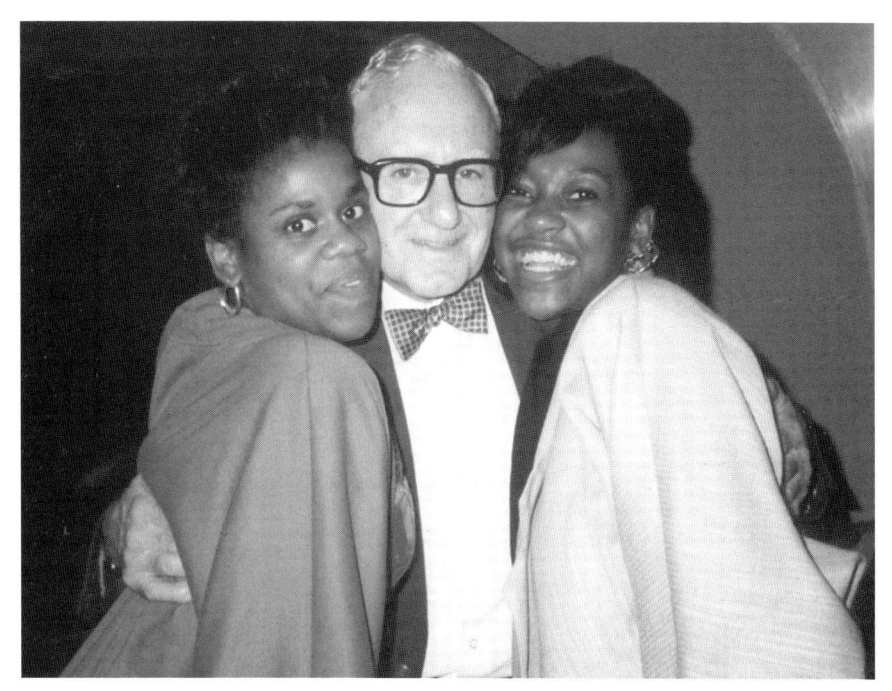

With my nurse and secretary in the VA Hospital

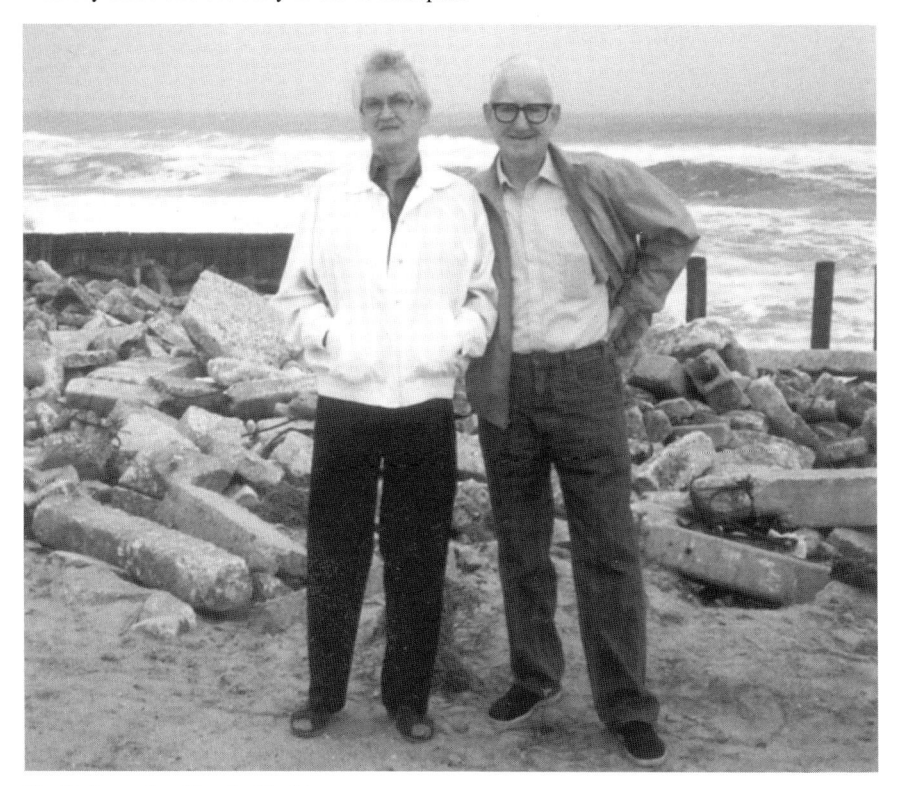

On St Augustine Beach, Florida

get himself back to Britain where he hoped to get a job in Wales, whence he came. I was left with the opportunity to go to Teheran fairly often. I had become very attached to Betty and the bus trip was well worthwhile.

Back in Ireland, Marie Bradley had cleared out the Belcoo home and had the two children and Gloria staying with her in Fintona.

An older sister was working in London and she came up with the bright idea of taking Gloria with her to London and getting her lessons in typing and then a job there. Six weeks of that was enough for Gloria and she went back to Ireland. She apparently got a small apartment in Belfast and remained there. Marie brought the children up to visit her every once in a while. Her drinking problems did not improve, but apparently she made some attempt to get help.

When I visited my mother in 1962, she told me that she had turned on the television one evening, looking at the Belfast channel. There was Gloria being interviewed on an Alcoholics Anonymous or some other alcoholic rehabilitation programme. Gloria was admitting the whole story about her drinking and her drugging and how she had ruined her marriage and her family. My mother nearly went through the floor. She had no idea of how bad things were until she saw Gloria telling the true story on television. However, I am ahead of myself.

I got to know a lot of the staff at Amman & Whitney, the Greeks, Americans, Indians, South Americans, Filipinos, etc., in the head office in Teheran and up and down the line. Usually nobody ever passed my hospital without coming in to say 'Hello' or give me a letter. Betty sent notes and supplies down, the bearers of which I got to know very well. Some would stay overnight when I got the hospital open, as we had inpatients' beds which were never needed, so we became like a little hotel along the road. This brightened things up and we were always glad to see somebody coming by to spend an evening. We made sure we never got caught again without some hospitable 'libations'.

My story got to be well known and the Americans, practically all of whom had been divorced in the past, advised me that that was the only route to go. Dr Flamank agreed and of course Betty, who had been divorced some years earlier, was of the same opinion. She wrote to a friend of hers in Nevada whom she had known in Spain and asked him how I should go about it. He replied, 'The only way to go is to Reno. Live there six weeks, get your divorce and get out.' As I shall tell later, that was not as easy as it sounded.

As the summer passed, we got better used to the way of life and the time did not drag at any stage. The weekends that I did not go to Teheran, Clive and I went to Hamadan and sometimes dropped in to the Morrison Knudsen camp. The second-rate hotel down from the Bou Ali had concerts nearly every night and we would meet other Europeans and Americans there. We had some very enjoyable evenings.

We would go down in the ambulance, park it in the hospital, and do the town on foot. Sometimes when we got back to the Bou Ali we would meet more English speakers from various other projects which were in Iran, other than road-building. There were service personnel from the air force and the army as the Shah was having his army trained by the Americans, and probably some British. We ran into Dutch, French and German businessmen, so by and large we had quite a lot of company and some good friends to break up the monotony.

Our houseboy was a very diligent worker and very anxious to ingratiate himself, and he kept the hospital very clean. I noticed that when he swept out the hospital he used a bunch of fine sticks tied together with some kind of string. It reminded me of what was used in Ireland when I was a child, it was something called a besom. Besom men travelled the country in Ireland selling besoms, which were bunches of heather with a handle driven through them. The heather was cut to a length of about a foot and a half and wrapped around a handle made of a stick which they smoothed off.

Our houseboy was stooping to sweep with his bunch of sticks with no handle. I went to the engineering department and got a piece of wood which would do for a handle, brought it back and showed him how to use it with his sticks without having to stoop. He seemed very impressed, and while I was there he swept out the hospital with the handle. A few days later I walked in and found him holding the broom by the lower end and stooping as usual. I guess he was too old a dog to whom to teach new tricks. I pulled the handle from the besom and let him do things his own way.

7

Where Next?

Although my life was getting more interesting and there were more events occurring from day to day, more patients and things to do in the evenings, I still found myself preoccupied with events at home in Ireland which I could not really forget. I was getting letters from friends, the occasional letter from Gloria and letters from her sister Marie.

I gave long thought to the avenues open to me.

My first consideration was my children, as I had now accepted the fact that Gloria, my wife, was a lost cause. Not having been able to straighten her out while I was living with her, there was no way I could ever redeem her by going back and trying to make a living with her as a millstone around my neck. Going back to Ireland would leave me in a dire predicament. I had no home and would have nowhere to live. My children were living with their aunt and my wife was living God knows where. I could not have a car because my insurance was defunct. I might get insurance at an exorbitant rate, but without a job, as Northern Ireland was now a closed shop, no car, no home or home address, this was the last consideration of the equation.

Secondly, I could consider going to my father with hat in hand and offering to help him out and maybe inherit the practice. Had this choice been open, I reasoned that if my father had had much sympathy with my situation he would have offered it to me earlier. My mother had suggested some such solution to my problems but my father was of the opinion that I drank too much and was too popular with the drinking crowd for him to jeopardize his practice by bringing me in. This was not to say that he did not drink himself – he did. He liked to drink, and most evenings when he came in after work he had had a glass of punch with my mother before he went to bed for as long as I could remember. My mother was the daughter of an alcoholic father and she could drink anybody under the table. She proved this on occasions when we were at functions. She could tell me the next morning how I had overindulged, although we drank drink for drink until such time as I couldn't remember where I went off the rails until she told me. So I thought my father had not really given me a fair break. Although we were friendly he really never forgave me until he died and he confirmed his disapproval by cutting me and my brother Kevin completely out of his will.

The third alternative would be to take a job as an assistant physician in England. It would be easy to get car insurance again, although expensive, but as an assistant I would have been supplied with a car and housing. I would have to do the worst 'scut work' part of the practice no matter who I worked for, and I would again have had to take Gloria and the children to live with me.

The fourth alternative was to go to the United States and get a divorce, as the Americans had advised me to do. Before I could do that, I would have to get an immigration visa to the United States. After that, to practice medicine in the United States, and to get an internship or residency, I had to pass the ECFMG examination. This was the Educational Council for Foreign Medical Graduates, which had been established in 1957 or 1958 – at least, that is when I first heard about it.

When I graduated in 1949 it was considered by one of the 'grinders' who crammed students in Dublin that anyone passing the final examination anywhere in Ireland would have no problem passing a state examination in the United States. At that time an immigrant doctor who wanted to work in one of the states took the state examination, and if he passed he could take an internship, a residency or whatever he could get. When it was completed he could hang up his shingle, or nameplate. Many of the graduates in my year had done that. They had specialized, or gone into general practice, and they had all done well. I only knew one who returned, and he came back because he was too lazy to do weekends and night work.

After a lot of consideration, many sleepless nights and many walks around Avej by myself, thinking and turning over the various alternatives in my mind and asking God to advise me, I came to the lonely decision that the ECFMG and immigration to America was the best of my rotten choices. My love for Gloria, a lot of which, I began to realize, was pity, was beginning to fade and turn sour. It came home to me that my Irish failure was not all my own and on my lonely meditation on my predicament I realized that before I had become involved with Gloria I had been pretty successful. Now that I had got away from her I was beginning to save money, practise good medicine, make good friends, drink less and by and large the outlook for my future was beginning to brighten.

Looming over the picture, however, was a grey shadow, and that was my Catholic religion.

Catholicism in Ireland, for the poorest and most ignorant peasant and lowest slum dweller up to the most highly educated and highly cultured professional university graduate, was a fear of God, doom and disaster which would be visited upon the sinner. Preached from the pulpit in country chapels and city cathedrals was the theme that those who went against the church teachings on birth control, marriage, and subscription and financial support of the church would have misfortunes, accidents and catastrophes. These would not only befall them in the next world but in the immediate future. Missioners came to the churches and gave retreats, and many stories were told of straying Catholics who suffered disasters as the result of neglecting their clergy and the Catholic way of life. I had come to believe that I should not even fly in a plane without first confessing to my priest and taking off with a clear conscience as the result of absolution.

After living in Iran for some months and not having had an opportunity to attend Mass or confession, I realized that misfortune had not overtaken me, and I began to see that my neglect of my Catholic duties had no effect at all on the outcome of my life. It came home to me that divorce would be worth the risk, and the resultant excommunication from the Catholic Church would be tolerable and might even bring an improvement in my circumstances by not being a factor in my decisions.

I realized that I could deal directly with God, and since then the clerical middle man has played no part in my religious or secular life. Having cleared that hurdle, the rest of my decisions were the result of reasoning and the choice of the best paths to take towards my future, unencumbered by superstition.

I got in touch with the ECFMG in Evanston, Illinois, where they were then based, and within two weeks I got all the facts about the ECFMG examination. They even sent me a sample of a multiple choice examination, which was the method used by the ECFMG to entitle foreign medical graduates to apply for residencies and internships in the United States.

I could get English updated medical books written by Americans which instructed how to take the examination. They did not teach with a view to a multiple choice examination, but in subsequent years multiple choice textbooks became available by the dozen.

The next ECFMG examination was in September 1960 and could be taken in Teheran. I applied, and presented myself, having obtained time off through Dr Flamank. I studied my medical books out in the desert, thinking that I had done pretty well.

At the University in Teheran the examination started at eight in the morning. The first half would take three hours, with 150 questions. The second half would take place after lunch, with another three hours and 150 questions. After that there would be an English test to find out if the candidate's English was of a high enough standard to be admitted to the United States.

I started the examination leisurely. There was a question followed by five answers. One blacked out the space opposite the answer one thought was the correct one. Some of the questions were not strictly medical and were not of practical value, for example, the percentage of mortality and morbidity from various diseases, biochemical questions and questions on physiology and anatomy. By and large, the whole examination was a surprise and it certainly was an education. When the three-hour period was up, I had about 30 questions unanswered. The papers were taken and we were advised to be back at one o'clock to take the second half.

After lunch I went back to take the second half, and there was some delay. By two o'clock we had still not been given the question-and-answer sheets, and the proctor told us that some of the papers had been stolen and that the examination could not begin until they were returned.

By three o'clock they had not been returned, so I went to the proctor telling him that I could not wait any longer because I had to be back at work and catch a bus out of town. He was very kind and apologetic. He said he would register my complaint and have the examination annulled so that I could take it again in March. This was fortunate, because even if I got full marks in the second half I now know that I would have failed miserably on my morning attempt, due to my inexperience with multiple choice exams. Six weeks later, I was notified by the ECFMG authorities that I had a clean sheet and could take the examination the next time as if it were my first. One was allowed three failures, after which the examination could not be taken again ever. Three failures would be exclusion from the possibility of ever getting into the United States to practise medicine.

It was now time to start working on my immigration visa into the United States. The American Embassy was across the street just down from the Amman & Whitney office. I went there and put in an application. I had to make several visits to the embassy and I found the elderly ladies working there to be quite unfriendly and brusque. This was my experience later at other embassies in West Africa, and I presumed that American Embassy staff's first interest was to discourage immigrants to the United States through legal channels.

After having chest X-rays, physical examinations and filling forms and getting references, I was finally told to come in the following week and my green card would be ready. It took years for me to realize what a precious and life-changing event it was to get a green card for immigration into the United States.

With the advent of autumn Iran was beginning to cool down, and Avej had the occasional cool breeze although the sunshine continued. Parvis brought me and my driver on a hunt for mountain goats and mountain sheep in the rugged mountains north of Avej. He supplied rifles and brought food for a picnic at midday. I had known these mountain goats were pretty nimble on their feet but I found that when one hunted them one needed to be nimble also. The trails we followed took steep routes around the sides of mountains and there were places where I was definitely afraid I was going to fall and break my neck. Some of these paths were only the width of my foot.

My driver had not much experience of this type of hunting either and made known to me that he did not feel safe and he would like to return to the ambulance, which we had brought to the foot of the hills. I agreed that I had had enough of this after about three hours' climbing. Parvis told us that we could go back and he would see us later. Going back was as dangerous as going up, especially as we ended up in some cul-de-sacs where we had taken the wrong path. I definitely felt panic at times and, had I not had my driver with me to encourage me, I might certainly have been stuck up that mountain for the night.

We finally got back to the ambulance and we were very glad to get back to the camp in Avej and have a stiff drink. When Clive heard of our adventures he laughed heartily and was glad he had not been invited.

I had some extra time in Teheran as the ambulance was beginning to show signs of wear and tear and needed quite a bit of service. Even the shock absorbers gave out, making travel on the rough roads a really rocky experience. Some garage mechanic had discovered that jeep shock absorbers fitted the Volkswagen ambulances and had fitted them in anticipation of longer life. It made the ride very rough. After about two months the shock absorbers survived, but one of them pulled a lump out of the chassis of the ambulance, which meant six weeks without any kind of transport. The engineer was very helpful and when we needed to go to Hamadan he brought us in the evening and we could go back with him the following day.

Progress on the roads seemed to be going nowhere, but not knowing anything about roadwork, we were surprised when suddenly about 10 miles of what looked like hopeless dust and dirt was suddenly surfaced, making the trip to Hamadan much more comfortable and quicker. It brought back my belief in American road building and reminded me that during the war, in a bog in the west of Ireland, an enormous American plane had come down. The local people thought it was going to be there for ever as it was at least 5 miles into the bog. The crew, or the airmen, in the plane were interned in the Republic because it was neutral, but somehow permission had been granted for the Americans to get their plane out. They came in and in three weeks they had built a road through what had seemed an impenetrable bog. They got the plane taken apart and onto transporters and had it all out and back to Northern Ireland in three weeks. A blind eye was turned to neutrality, but I am sure there was not a family within 10 miles of the downed plane that didn't have relatives in the United States. The German defeat was within sight anyway, and Germany had too many fish to fry to pay attention to a breach of neutrality by Ireland.

The road between Avej and Teheran was also improving and after 20 miles going north was plain sailing, either in the ambulance or in the bus.

The bus trips were interesting because anything could be taken on the bus, from tethered goats to chickens and sheep with their legs tied. The bus stopped at every *chai-khana* on the way, with a long stop in Ghazvin, a large city, where the food was quite good. The buses did break down on occasions, being mostly very old, probably pre-war. They were Mercedes Benz buses and, living up to their reputation, never did I see one that couldn't be repaired and continue the trip. Fan belts seemed to be the biggest problem and probably if the buses had been properly serviced they would have never broken down.

I felt I was accomplishing something as I had a green card and I was involved with the ECFMG examination and knew what I was in for. There was no way I could study for the examination, because the medical textbooks that I was using did not include the basic sciences, which were a large part of the ECFMG, or statistics, which were of little value in the everyday practice of medicine, surgery or obstetrics. I had decided not to take the examination again in Iran but to wait until I arrived back in civilization and got access to appropriate medical literature. I had also heard that there were correspondence courses to help one to pass the ECFMG, but I was not in the position to get started on such a course, living in the desert.

8

Winter and a Decision

As the summer passed, the clinic was getting quite busy, with a lot of the local peasants and occasional workers being seen. Nobody was very ill but the locals coming around the clinic reminded me of dispensaries in Ireland and my surgeries in Tyrone and Fermanagh. There were children with sore throats and colds, women with colds and abdominal pains, and men with pains in their backs, headaches, sore feet, corns, ingrowing toenails etc.

After my experience on the house call to see the woman with the appendicitis, I never even dared to examine any of the women who came to the clinic, but treated them on history alone. The workers were usually genuinely ill, with cuts which we sutured, and bruises, and most accident injuries were the result of trauma on the road. These we were able to treat successfully.

One man was brought in on whom a crane had fallen. He was semi-conscious and there was no way we could treat him in our hospital. We got him into the ambulance and had a message sent up to Dr Flamank via the radio, and he told us he would meet us at the office. After a long drive we got there about seven or eight in the evening and the office was closed. We had difficulty in getting in touch with anybody. Finally, another ambulance arrived, picked up the patient and he was taken away. Arrangements had been made apparently and he did not return during my time in the camp. I never saw him again.

Towards the end of September the weather was getting cooler and one could feel autumn in the air. We had to get warmer clothes and wear our jackets. We bought long johns, Iranian-style, made of cotton. We could buy them in Hamadan or even in Avej, where there were vendors selling them on the streets. They were blue and white stripes and all types of colours. During the summer I saw men wearing nothing else except these long johns. Looking back, they seemed like an early form of jump suit. However, they were warm. We had to put the heat on in the hospital and to keep pestering the contractor to keep our tank filled with oil. Snow flurries grew into snowfalls and in November it was just frost every night.

One night, coming from Hamadan with supplies in the ambulance, we had severe problems because the snow falling on the windscreen was freezing as it fell and the wiper could not get it off. We went into a *chai-khana* and got a salt cellar and shook salt on the windscreen. That worked for a while, but as we got along the road even that didn't work. On the long climb up to Avej we had to get out every half-mile to scrape the windscreen. To crown our misery, when we got back to the hospital the houseboy was gone and there was no heat or light. We eventually found somebody in the contractor's building to get something started, but he told us our oil was low and it only gave us enough heat to carry us through the night. We were completely dependent on the oil heater and the electric blower.

The following day I called Teheran and they told us if we had no heat we would have to go and stay in the Bou Ali Hotel in Hamadan. I went over to the contractor's office to find that he had gone to Teheran and had left a skeleton crew behind. Apparently, with the snowfall, roadwork could not be continued so they had discharged most of the employees. It was now getting towards the end of November and there were snowfalls every other day, with drifts along the sides of the road. Passing trucks and buses was a hazard because the road was not wide enough, and when we saw a truck in the distance the trick was to get to a wide part of the road and wait until it passed, then get as far as we could before the next oncoming truck. Travelling in the ambulance was now a difficult job and what was a slow trip before was now even slower because of snow and ice.

We decided to pack up as much as we could and head for the hotel. There we got in touch with Dr Flamank. He advised us to move into the Hamadan hospital the following day. The only really warm place we could get into was our ambulance. It had a very good heater, which Volkswagens were noted for.

As Avej was the most northerly hospital the predicament of snow closing everything down had not been anticipated. Rather than have us all up in Teheran waiting for the weather to clear, Dr Flamank's suggestion was that we move down the line. This would keep Mr Sherman off his back asking why they were paying doctors when there was nothing for them to do.

Rather than do this, Clive and I returned to our hospital in Avej with the driver early in the morning to see what could be done. We couldn't get the electricity started and nobody was there to fix the oil heater in the hospital so I had to return to the hospital in Hamadan. The ice and snow were the worst I had ever seen in my life. There were some areas along the road where the telephone wires were broken down with the ice and there was no communication whatsoever.

I was not getting any help from Teheran and I wasn't feeling well. I decided that I was not going to get much better down the line as I had no treatment and no doctor, so I decided to go to Teheran and told Dr Flamank so. He had the engineer arrange for a flight from Hamadan to Teheran and I left Clive and the driver and flew north.

When I got to Teheran Dr Flamank agreed with my diagnosis of probably pneumonia. He had me X-rayed and that confirmed it.

Betty decided that she would nurse me and got me to her apartment, where there was plenty of heat. She had an army cot with a lot of blankets. Dr Flamank brought some tetracycline and cough mixture and I settled down with the radio and some books that Betty got me, to hibernate until I got over the pneumonia. It took me ten days to recover and get over the cough. I probably had pleurisy, because I had pain in one side every time I breathed, but it gradually improved.

Dr Flamank began to talk again about my going further down the line, helping out Dr Turner and some of the doctors in Pol-i-doktar, where there was no snow and it was warmer. I was not enthusiastic about this idea and decided that I would get out of Iran. I had my green card, and Betty at this time agreed to leave with me and go back to the United States, where she had previously lived. She had a green card and said she would come with me and show me the ropes. I was by this time in love with Betty and had no doubt that when I was free I would marry her, so Reno and divorce was a must of first importance.

I tendered my resignation as I had now done a year's work with the Plan Organization, and as there was really no work to do nobody really objected to my leaving.

Betty also resigned, but her departure was differently received than mine. From Mr Sherman down to the drivers and the most insignificant employees her departure caused great sorrow. During the years she had been working for Amman & Whitney she had endeared herself to everyone with whom she had come in contact. I felt sorry for the doctors who would be down the line looking for supplies and the luxuries that Betty was able to send them. I knew that no successor would be as kind, thoughtful and sympathetic as Betty was.

For Betty and me the last two weeks were busy. The Armenian drivers and employees, who all appeared to be one family and related to each other, had parties every night for Betty, and as they knew what the relationship was between her and me, I was included. They brought us to their homes and to their parents' homes and to sheebeens around Teheran that we had never heard about. I drank more Russian vodka than I thought existed and I found that these Armenians enjoyed their drinking as much as any Irishman. They could dance and sing and make a lot of fun, as I had never had before or since. They always got us home safely and never left us until we were at the door.

The day before we left Iran one of the Armenians who had the use of a helicopter, owned by a rubber company in Teheran, brought us for a helicopter jaunt around the city. It was a very small helicopter and only held the pilot and two passengers. I will never forget that joyride because that was what it was. The most hair-raising experience was when the pilot switched off the engine and let us go into free fall. I understand this is a very dangerous thing to do but he was pretty adept and enjoyed our terror no end. Having no doors on the helicopter added to the experience.

The following morning we were seen off at the airport by every Armenian who was available. The goodbyes were sad and tearful and they gave Betty some beautiful and valuable souvenirs of Iran, which we still treasure.

The wait for the plane was short and soon we were aboard. The Armenians waved to us until we went through the last door. The plane was a Comet with three seats on each side of the aisle. I had a window seat and Betty was in the middle because I was still excited by flying and being able to see out. The plane took off eastwards and swung around at the edge of the city of Teheran to go westward. There was a great view of the city as it was a clear day and Mount Damávand looked beautiful in the morning sunshine. We had a great view and I realized how far the city of Teheran extended beyond where I had ever travelled. Looking back, I can now remember how few high-rise buildings there were and how Middle Eastern the city looked. There were very few trees and there was snow on the Elburz mountains. Where there was no snow it was brown earth. As we flew west and gained altitude we were soon in the clouds. That was my last view of Teheran.

I understand that now Teheran has many high-rise buildings and has become a very Western-appearing city. I always remember, however, how wide the streets were compared to what I had experienced at that time.

The thought of the future was exciting and I was looking forward to meeting Betty's parents and seeing the Isle of Wight, about which I had heard so much. Getting to America was also an exciting thought as I knew my future was there and I would finally escape and shake off the shackles of my earlier life. Having beautiful Betty along with me ready to throw in her lot made my doubtful future well worth the risk and all the brighter.

We arranged for a rental car to be available when we arrived in London. Betty had our tickets from London to San Francisco arranged before we left Teheran. That sort of thing was part of her job there. We were going from London to New York, where I would immigrate, and then continuing to San Francisco. This would give us two weeks at Betty's home in the Isle of Wight with her parents. There I would find a home from home, making friends for a lifetime. Most of them were Betty's friends and relatives and at the time of writing this we seem to have outlived them all.

It was daylight when we arrived in London, about three in the afternoon, and our car, a Morris Minor, was waiting for us. Everything we had in the world was with us and it all fitted into the car as it was a station wagon. We drove into London, where Betty had arranged rooms in the Cumberland Hotel. The porter was from Ireland, County Kerry, and when I gave him a 5-shilling tip he was our friend for life. That was a lot of money in those days. He told me to tell them to send Kelly when I was leaving.

The next day we went shopping in London and I bought two new suits, sports coats, slacks, shirts, shoes etc. What I had arrived with from Iran I gave to Mr Kelly when I left. I had never bought more than one suit at a time in my life and the one I gave to Kelly I had bought for my sister Dervilla's wedding seven years earlier. It was getting somewhat frayed around the edges. The shirts my mother had sent to me from Ireland I had nearly worn out, and the khaki uniforms I had been wearing in Iran I had left to my male nurse. I spent more in Austin Reed that day on clothes than I had spent since I first married Gloria.

Betty did some shopping and in the evening we had a Chinese dinner in Soho.

In the morning we set out for the Isle of Wight and we were soon in the country. I was seeing the south of England for the first time. The weather was dull and cold. For lunch it was my first experience of a real English pub and I was very impressed. The road was very civilized, well marked, well surfaced and wide. Iran was beginning to seem like a dream. When we reached Lymington we had timed it so that we were able to drive right onto the ferry for the Isle of Wight. It was now getting dark and the ferry was quite an experience for me. The island looked like a light on the horizon and finally we docked. There was a bar on the ferry and it was great to get some really good English draught beer. Driving off the ferry at Yarmouth, I was beginning to wonder whether Betty's parents would approve of me or not and I had some mixed feelings, to put it mildly.

* * *

When we arrived at 'Freshfield', Betty's parents' home, her mother came out to greet us and it was a very emotional and joyful meeting. I liked Betty's parents immediately. Her father was a very quiet man of few words but I knew I was welcome by his firm handshake and pleasant smile. We were all to become great friends before Betty and I left for the United States. Down through the years 'Freshfield' was more of a home to me than anything I have experienced since my departure from my parents' home in 1950.

That evening Betty and her mother got together a mixed grill, and this was my first good hearty English meal of bacon, eggs, sausages, thick lamb chops, English bread and butter with lots of strong tea with milk. What a change from Iran. After we had eaten, Betty and her father and I went into Newport to a pub, where we had a few beers and a chat. Her father was not up to drinking much as he had been in poor health for some years.

I was very impressed by my first experience of the Isle of Wight. During the next few days we toured the island, visiting Betty's uncle, who had been instrumental in getting her into the Royal Navy, and we visited her aunts, uncles and cousins. She introduced me to her solicitor in Newport, who was to be a great help to us in future years. He was so informal and friendly and the whole island was so easy-going it was like being in the west of Ireland, far away from the maddening throng.

There was a girl who used to deliver the newspapers, do favours and help out Betty's parents, and she volunteered to bring us to the local 'fun' pub one night, and she did. This was my first introduction to darts and to the hilarity of a really good friendly pub called The Sportsmen. Pat introduced us to all the regulars, one of whom was her boyfriend. We met his brother, his brother's wife and they introduced us to more people. They invited us to go on a pub crawl the next night. This introduced us to a way of life that was really fun. When I look back on it they were the best days of my life. Whenever we returned to the island, on vacations, or between jobs, or for whatever reason, we could go on a pub crawl and be sure to meet people we knew in every pub on the circuit.

As the Wight was an island, the distance one could go was limited. Betty being a native, and her father popular and very well known all over the island, having been a bit of a hellion in his youth, made us all the more easily accepted by the islanders. They did not usually take kindly to the 'overners', meaning people from the mainland.

We met an old friend of Betty's who had been a friend of her father's, a retired bank manager nicknamed Lofty. Lofty was a fund of jokes and stories and reminiscences and was great company. We used to meet him in the mornings in a pub called The Falcon. He introduced us to and had us join the Conservative Club in Newport, where we were sure to meet him any morning we were at a loose end or shopping in the town. He wasn't a native of the island but he had been there so long that he was accepted. As he was such a character, the islanders probably forgot that he was an overner. He could put on the Hampshire accent or the Yorkshire or London accent and told stories in different dialects so convincingly that he probably would have been a great actor if he had been so inclined.

The time on the island flew by, and as the time to go to Nevada, where I was bound for my divorce, grew nearer, I began to get lonely for the island. But the excitement about seeing the United States for the first time offset the impending loss of the fun and kindness of the island people.

I was beginning to be more apprehensive as I got closer to taking the big step of divorcing Gloria. I had yet to shake off the deeply ingrained conscious and subconscious fear of abandoning Catholicism and turning my back on all that my Catholic upbringing stood for. I knew I would be excommunicated but I also knew, after my time in Iran, that I would not experience sudden disaster by practising Christianity other than the Catholic style. Looking around me in Iran I had seen Muslims succeeding and in England I saw Protestants succeeding and I knew that in the United States Catholics were a small proportion of the population. Were I to go back to Ireland I would again be engulfed in Catholicism for breakfast, dinner and tea, seven days a week. Staying away would dilute the superstition and unwash the brainwash. I was determined also not to go from the frying pan into the fire by endorsing some other form of religion but to keep my options open and continue to avoid clergymen.

For this reason I did not even contact my parents, although I could have called them on the telephone. Betty and I thought that this divorce would have to be a surprise rather than give the opposition any chance to prepare a counter-attack before we had our ducks in line.

The day to depart drew near and we said goodbye to our friends and on the last day we bade sad farewells to Betty's parents, drove back to the ferry and back to London. We spent a night in the Cumberland and the following morning, after a hearty English breakfast, we drove to the airport, returned the car and we were back in the fast lane on our way to New York, San Francisco, Reno and to a surprisingly difficult divorce.

9

A Lengthy Divorce in Reno

The plane we flew on was a Boeing 707, a relatively new plane and to me an enormous monster that I thought would never get off the ground. We flew non-stop to New York, where we arrived in the afternoon, and I went through Immigration. The accents, the airport, New York, the piped music, all were a real wonder to me. Music in elevators and in banks took me a long time to get used to. Sliding doors which opened before you reached them caught me off guard. I put out my hand a few times to open the door and suddenly it opened away from me or slid away.

It was nice at Immigration to be welcomed to the United States by the officials as they saw me for the first time, knowing by my papers that I had not been there before.

After about two hours' wait we got back on the plane heading for San Francisco. We had had a meal on the transatlantic flight and now we had another while crossing the United States. I had not slept on the transatlantic crossing and now I had a window seat and could not stop looking out into the darkness trying to see America. We were flying at 32,000 feet, so there was nothing I could see.

Finally, it was announced that we were approaching San Francisco and it was a very impressive sight as the plane circled and approached the airport from the sea. We got a taxi into the city with all our possessions and by this time I was getting sleepy and definitely suffering from jet lag. We were eight hours behind European time and it was about midnight when we got to the hotel, which would have been eight in the morning Greenwich

Mean Time, and I had had very little sleep. I fell into bed regardless of jet lag or time until eight the next morning. On getting up I noticed that I was missing one bag, which contained all my medical books, but I felt it might have been mixed up with Betty's luggage and could be in her room.

I showered, shaved, dressed and went to knock on Betty's door. She was up, dressed and packing. My missing bag was not among hers. We called the airport and the taxi company but nobody had any idea of what had happened to it. It only contained books which would go out of date shortly so we gave up the search.

We had breakfast in the Francis Drake Hotel, where we had stayed that night, and went out to find the bus station and prepare to leave for Reno. We had time to explore San Francisco, where Betty had lived and worked about ten years before and where she had met her former husband. We rode the streetcars up and down and it was all like fairyland to me. Betty was amused by my amazement and my ignorant wonderment.

We went to a bank and changed traveller's cheques into dollars. One of my great surprises was to hear the piped music in the bank. To me, banks were the very serious and quiet establishments in Ireland and England. I had also noticed the piped music in the elevators in the hotel and all this accentuated to me that this was a different world. Americans were different and business establishments had not the sombre atmosphere that they had in Europe. It really took me a long time to get used to the piped music. It made me feel that while this went on serious business would not be conducted. I had often heard the saying that 'someone was left breathless', and now I understood what it meant. I was frequently breathless with what I saw in San Francisco and, later, the rest of America. The enormous cars, countless taxi-cabs, the crowds in the streets all in a hurry and the children driving cars, no horses or bicycles. In those days if one stepped off the pavement in San Francisco the traffic stopped even if one was not in a crosswalk. I was a jaywalker from way back, but when I stepped off the pavement in San Francisco intending to beat a car by running across the street, I was amazed that traffic in both directions stopped for me. I later found this to happen in Reno also. I have not been to the West for a long time and I do not know if that is still how things are.

During that day we made arrangements to catch an early bus to Reno the following morning. We went to a restaurant for lunch, where I had my first American hamburger. The waitress could not understand me so I turned the ordering over to Betty. For a long time I didn't order in a restaurant but let Betty do it. This was the first time I realized that I had a thick Irish accent which might have been understood on the East Coast but in the West it certainly was not.

The next morning we checked out of the hotel, and got a taxi to the bus station, and there again I was amazed at the number of buses and how different they looked from those in the British Isles. Our luggage was stowed underneath and we got aboard, where the seats were very comfortable.

It also surprised me that the bus had automatic transmission, something I had never seen before, except in an occasional car. In those days even the buses in Dublin and London were manual, using a clutch, so that the drive was erratic, bumping and crashing gears.

Soon we were at the outskirts of the city and I was also amazed by streets crossing over streets. The only bridges I had seen were bridges over railways or railway bridges over streets. Streets over streets I had never seen. Now I know them as overpasses. We were shortly out of the city and I saw my first four-lane highway. When we got on the open road the bus picked up speed and soon we were bounding along at what must have been 70 to 75 miles an hour. I just could not believe the way the road went for miles and miles, the long curves and hills winding as far as the eye could see. The bus stopped at some towns but the first big stop was Sacramento. There we had a chance to have a meal, a hamburger, of course. We did not wander far from the bus station as all our possessions were on the bus and if we missed that we were in trouble.

After Sacramento the four-lane highway gave way to two-lane, but it still seemed very wide to me, and later we got into the hills and mountains. The scenery changed with the pine trees and the long climbing hills and smaller towns with wooden buildings that really reminded me of cowboy movies I had seen. The last stop before Reno was Truckee. In those days there were no high-rise buildings in Reno, the highest being eight and twelve storeys. One was the Mapes Hotel and the other was a bank. We unloaded and counted our luggage, and stowed it in the bus station. We then went out to look for somewhere to stay. About five blocks from the bus station we found the Chamber of Commerce next door to the post office. Here we got lists of places we might stay, a map of Reno and telephone numbers of boarding houses. We called one and spoke to a pleasant lady who told us she had two rooms available.

This was our first contact with Abby and Pearl. We got a taxi to Hill Street, which was where they had their boarding house. One was a Texan and the other was a Virginian. Pearl, the Texan, showed us the rooms and I got a small narrow room with a single bed and bare necessities across the hall from a bathroom. Betty got a larger room next door, on the corner, and with more windows than mine, but that was the least of my worries. I had somewhere to store my things.

Again, I was impressed by the heating. There were radiators in the rooms and these were hot. I had gone to school in Dublin, where the radiators were supposed to heat the school but they were never more than warm. We used to sit on them and warm our backsides. But at Abby's and Pearl's you could not touch them, they were almost red-hot. Occasionally the steam hissed out but they certainly warmed the rooms. Outside it was frosty and cold, much colder than in San Francisco, so we got out our warm clothes and prepared for a long stay in Reno, little knowing how much longer it was going to be than we had anticipated.

Abby and Pearl laid down their laws. There was no question of hanky-panky, such as staying late in each other's rooms. Every night had to be spent in the home because when my divorce came through, one of them would come to court and testify that I had lived six weeks in Nevada and that every night was spent there and not elsewhere. They were very impressed by the fact I was a doctor from Ireland and that Betty was English. We told them we had been in Iran. Betty impressed them because she had been in Australia and had been in America before and had lived in San Francisco. They promised to show us the area and Pearl said she would drive us to Lake Tahoe the following day.

Betty and I walked downtown, which was within walking

distance, about six blocks. I saw for the first time the permanent banner across the street in Reno, although I had seen it in movies, which says, 'The Biggest Little City in The World'. The casinos were staggering. Rows and rows of slot machines and people playing them, and keno, a kind of lottery, going day and night, like the bingo halls in the parishes in Ireland but much more sophisticated. There were amusements of all descriptions, food available, cafés, little restaurants, and amazement upon amazement. It was almost frightening what a difference this America was from anything I had ever known or could imagine.

I could now remember gangster movies and movies about millionaires and I could see that they were all really genuine and this was the way it was.

Having come from the Isle of Wight which had re-established my previous non-Iranian experience and nearly brought me back into thinking small-town, small country green fields, quietness etc., to be suddenly landed in this mad world gave strange feelings in the pit of my stomach. It made me realize that I had wasted the previous nine years in the bogs and the mountains of Tyrone and Fermanagh. Knowing nothing, seeing nothing, earning nothing and seeing nothing new, just going to seed, unaware that there was a big, mad, wild, active, teeming world outside which was passing me by. It brought home to me that my past was finished, that my quest was justified and that ever again living with Gloria would be impossible, unthinkable and must be forgotten.

That night alone in my little dark room it was almost impossible to sleep. I had a lot of thinking to do and a lot of sadness and some regrets. However, I knew I would have to bear my regrets but never give in to the thought of going back to Ireland. There was no possibility that I could leave the children with Gloria but planning to take them would have to wait until after the divorce had been completed.

As I got over the jet lag I began to sleep better and we became friendly with other occupants of 220 Hill Street. Ray was a New Yorker, Kay was an English lady from Iowa and they were fun people, also on the road to divorce. There was an elderly lady called Mrs Bush, who was the housekeeper in the Mapes Hotel. She had a forbidding attitude until we got to know her. She was a permanent resident at the boarding house and a very kind woman who became a great friend until we left, and long after until we lost touch.

Kay had a car so she, Ray and Betty and I had some excursions into the countryside, including Virginia City, which was another fantastic place. It was just the same as it had been during the gold rush days, with all kinds of exciting museums and bars and restaurants. There were memorabilia of Mark Twain, who had lived there, Charles Dickens, who had visited there, and especially Boot Hill Cemetery.

We visited Sparks, on the other side of Reno, which had casinos and was on a smaller scale than Reno. It had some very good restaurants, including one good Chinese. We visited Pyramid Lake which was nearby, drove through the desert and generally got to know the area very well.

Just around the corner from our boarding house was a bar run by 'the Deacon'. He was a very funny and droll man. Ray had the knack of saying things that irritated the Deacon, who had a black moustache, black hair and was probably Greek, but irritated or not he was a very funny man. He had what seemed to me many funny American sayings because I was only beginning to learn American.

Betty and I were doing our best to live as cheaply as we could, pooling our resources, but one night we came in rather late with Ray and Kay. We had been having a few drinks at the Deacon's and there was a light under Mrs Bush's door. Ray had a flat bottle of bourbon and we decided to visit Mrs Bush. She had given Ray a job in the Mapes Hotel and his divorce was about to come through, so he wanted to suggest to her that I get his job. He offered Mrs Bush a drink, which she accepted. She got out some glasses and we all sat on her bed, and soon we had her laughing and relating stories about her trips to Tucson, Arizona. She said Tucson was the only place to live and she knew the West very well. She was the salt of the earth if ever there was such.

The next day she was back to her own stern self and went off to work with just a 'Hi', and no mention of the night before. On my second day in Reno I had visited Betty's friend's friend, the Judge. He was very polite but said that he was not in a position, being a judge, to recommend that I attend any particular attorney in Reno. He did say I should go and speak to a group of attorneys in town and they could recommend someone to me. I did that and I was appointed to a younger attorney who seemed quite friendly. I gave him all my information, together with $250. He did say that my wife not being there and not being available might delay my divorce, but he got her address and made arrangements to have the divorce papers served to her. In Ireland, the only person who could deliver them would be a local policeman and arrangements were made for that to be done.

I had not been corresponding with Gloria since I was in Iran and so this was going to be a surprise and would break my cover.

In two weeks I had letters pouring in. The first one was from Gloria, telling me how heartbroken she was, how she couldn't believe I was going to do this and that her brother Seamus when he heard the news had slapped her face. He had told her that she should have told him sooner and would not believe that she did not know it was about to happen.

Next day there was a letter from my father, telling me that he hoped I knew what I was doing and reminding me that this would mean excommunication from the Catholic Church. He also told me that Gloria's brother had telephoned him and said they would have to fight this divorce and that they could put their money together to have an attorney in Reno fight the case. My father had told him he must be crazy and that by no means would he take sides against his own son on the side of the brother-in-law who had done nothing but give me problems; that my wife had given me problems and her family had done nothing for her until they found her handed back into their care. My father told me it was my own life and that he would always love me no matter what way it went and that my mother stood by him. Afterwards, I often thought that the letter was written by my father, but the ideas were my mother's. However it was, it made no difference to our relationship and they stood by me and never criticized me from that day on.

Looking back, it surprised me that not one relative ever said I was wrong or I should do other than I did.

Gloria's sister Marie wrote to me and asked me to discontinue my plan, and another sister wrote to ask me to write to Gloria, but I never again wrote a line to her. It was a complete break with no regrets but with many sorrows.

Ray finally completed his divorce and left and went back to New York. By now I realized that, unlike Ireland or England, living without a car was impossible. Pearl had brought us up to Lake Tahoe and shown us the surrounding countryside and this was a long trip. We were getting tired of walking around Reno and taking a bus to Sparks and then waiting for hours to get back. We took a bus to Virginia City, and that was a day's outing because we could not get back until night.

I saw a car advertised, in mint condition, in Sparks for $150. I went out and interviewed the salesmen and asked them what mileage it got per gallon. They looked at each other and laughed. Mileage per gallon in those days meant nothing. Petrol was so cheap. The car was a 1948 four-door Chevrolet, looked very good and drove quite well, so that was the end of public transport, such as it was. I was getting Americanized. Having a car opened up new vistas and with the weather getting warmer and the days getting longer, we were really able to explore the surrounding countryside.

Soon after Ray had obtained his divorce and left, Kay also got hers and left to return to Iowa in her car, which she had driven to Reno. Betty and I were now left to our own devices and we got to know Mrs Bush much better. She offered me a job in the Mapes Hotel as the linen delivery man.

I was delighted, and the next day I went with her to work in the basement at the Mapes. There was a laundry there and all the bed linen was washed, dried and folded then packed away on shelves. My job was to get a large dolly with wheels and fill it with the sheets etc. that were needed on the floors, then bring it up on the elevator and fill the linen closets on each floor. There were two closets on each floor and there had to be linen in them at all times. I got in early, before the maids arrived and before the rooms were vacated, to get the linen in ready for the maids to make up the beds. No sooner had I filled the closets on one floor than I had to move on to the next. When I was out of linen I had to take the elevator to the basement and fill up again, repeating the process all day. By the time I had reached the twelfth floor it was time to go back and start again on the fourth, or whichever floor a call came from that the closets were empty. I soon got the knack of it and found out which floors needed the most linen, and I knew from the occupation roster where the most rooms were occupied. When I got into the routine it was not a difficult job but it was tiring pushing the dolly around the corridors and sometimes having to make an emergency delivery carrying the linen in my arms and using the stairs. I was not allowed to use an elevator in which there were guests.

There was a free staff cafeteria in the basement and there were showers which I could use in the morning and after work. I was paid 90 cents an hour at the end of the week and tax was being withheld.

Betty's first application for a job was as secretary with a lady attorney and she got the job immediately. With both of us working, the time began to pass more quickly, and now having transport we were able to take trips on weekends to Tahoe, Virginia City and even one weekend to visit an old friend of Betty's in Tonapah, which was almost halfway to Las Vegas. It was late in the afternoon when we arrived and we met Betty's friend. His name was Rocky and he was a mining engineer who had a gold mine, and he brought us down the mine to see the gold being mined. At that time the price of gold was controlled – it was figured at around $35 an ounce – and they smelted it and made it into gold bars. If the bar was too heavy they got a hacksaw and cut some of it off. They then sent it through the mails. It was quite safe because of the controlled price of gold. Seeing the large boiling cauldron of gold was fascinating and the attitude towards gold made it seem quite worthless. This was quite a contrast from the precautions and the armed protection and searches which I saw years later in diamond mines in Africa, but I would say things changed when the control of the price of gold was discontinued.

On our first evening we had a great meal with Rocky and his

friends, eating huge steaks and drinking beer and whiskey as quickly as it could be put up. The following morning we did our tour of the mine and the smelting plant and my nerves at least were pretty well shattered and my head was splitting.

Driving in Nevada was another adventure. We were always warned never to run short of water and always carried lots of drinking water with us. It was considered much more serious to run out of water than to run out of petrol. The miles and miles of empty road with no traffic in either direction was reminiscent of Iran, except that in Iran there was more traffic and many trucks. We could travel for one to two hours in Nevada then and see no traffic or any sign of life.

Looking back on this, I see how naive we were to drive so far in a car that was an unknown quantity, but it did stand up well and never gave us any problems whatsoever. I soon got used to the loose steering but as long as the road was not rough and was well paved it did not cause any trouble.

On another weekend we ventured a trip to San Francisco via Sacramento. As we got closer to San Francisco, crossing some bridges with heavy traffic was nerve-racking. It was dark and all we could see was lights in the distance. Sometimes the steering began to vibrate and the only way to stop it was to slow down or stop and start again. This caused some irritation in the traffic which was following us but there was nothing else I could do. We got to San Francisco and saw the outskirts. We went to the beach and saw the places with which Betty was familiar. The scenery on the road between San Francisco and Sacramento and Reno was varied and beautiful.

As the six weeks from the time I had arrived in Reno drew near I went to visit my attorney, expecting that he had the date for my divorce, but he kept telling me there were delays. I visited again in two weeks and he put it off again and said that my in-laws had hired an attorney to fight the case and that he was stalling.

Because it seemed I was to be in Reno longer than expected, I applied for a job as a lab man in the local hospital, which paid $2 per hour. I knew I could do this quite easily as I had worked in labs all through my medical school. I got an appointment with the lady in charge of hiring employees. I got time off and before lunch rushed over to the hospital expecting to be seen as soon as I went in. I was shown into a room with no other applicants, and after waiting 45 minutes I tried to find out who I was supposed to see. The secretary told me it was Sister so and so, a nun. I waited another half an hour and was told that she had not arrived yet. I had to leave and go back to work. The following day I tried again and the secretary told me that as I had not waited to see Sister the day before she did not want to see me. Obviously, when she saw my CV she realized that I was an Irish Catholic looking for a divorce and that was the end of my chance for that job. I remained at the Mapes for 90 cents an hour.

The weeks dragged on into months and my attorney continued to stall and it was getting more difficult to get to see him. Betty told my sad story to her boss. Nada said that this was ridiculous and to get my file from my attorney and bring it to her and she would pick it up. The next time I got to see my attorney I told him I wanted to take my business elsewhere and he said, 'Okay, it will cost you two hundred and fifty dollars.' I had already paid him $250 and I told him so. He said he had put a lot of work into the case and gave me a long story, so I went and consulted with Betty and we got the money together, paid him off and moved my case over to Nada. It was now the end of August but Nada got on the ball and she got my divorce through in two weeks.

Abby and Pearl both came to court and vouched for my presence in Nevada for over six weeks. The opposing attorney put up a poor case and my divorce was granted.

We went down to a local bar where the girls used to swing on bars from the roof and we all celebrated. It was an amazing relief to know that we could leave Reno. That night we went out and celebrated with Mrs Bush. I gave notice at the Mapes Hotel and the following morning I collected my last cheque. We went to the Court House and Betty and I got married. We were ready for the high road to wherever else it led us.

10

Back to England

We packed the green Chevy with everything we owned and Betty had the good idea to get a long chain, which we looped through the handles of our luggage and padlocked it so that it couldn't be stolen. Early in the morning we filled up with petrol, checked battery and tyres and headed for Sparks and Highway 80, going due north to Lovelock, Winnemucka, Elkton and the Utah border.

One of the guests at 220 Hill Street had driven from New York and gave us a wedding present of his AAA Triptick*, which he had obtained before he left. He was going to fly back and that was the most useful thing we could have had as we did not have the faintest idea how to get to New York from Nevada.

Highway 80 was not four-lane in those days, it was two-lane, but we reached Salt Lake City the first night. The car gave no trouble and the next day we crossed the Rockies to Cheyenne, Wyoming, where we spent the night. The following night we stayed in Omaha, Nebraska. The change of scenery was impressive and magnificent.

On some part of the highway in Iowa at a toll booth the car stopped while we paid and would not move. We had to get towed to a garage. The mechanic said the car would be fixed by the next morning, so we stayed in a motel. True to his word, he was there at ten o'clock and the car was repaired. Apparently a timing chain had broken and he either repaired it or put on a new one, but the charge was very reasonable. He did advise me not to drive too fast

---

*A collection of route maps published by The American Automobile Association.

and I realized that that was what had caused the problem. We had been going 70 and 75 miles an hour in a very old car whose limitations I was not aware of. We took it easy from there on and arrived in Chicago two days later.

We had tickets on the *Queen Mary* sailing out of New York on 11 October, 1961 so we decided to do some touring on the way. We spent a day in Chicago and then headed east to Philadelphia, where we spent two days, and then on to New Jersey.

The Pennsylvania Turnpike was fascinating as it was four-lane and had limited access, something I had not seen before. There were also some tunnels through which the road passed, reminding me of the Mersey Tunnel in England.

We took the Garden State Parkway to Newark, New Jersey, and it was not busy in those days but much busier than any part of the road we had passed before. I had often seen photographs of the New York skyline and when I had flown in from London I did not get a good view of it. However, when I got the first glimpse away in the distance of the silhouette of Manhattan, it was a thrill to realize I was now actually seeing the real thing. I got the sensation of goose pimples that I sometimes felt when I got scared suddenly. It looked just like it did in the pictures. It was a very clear day and that was probably the clearest view of the Manhattan skyline I have ever had, and I have seen it many times since.

As we got nearer to New York the silhouette rose and became bigger until it was constantly occupying the horizon from the Newark area. Betty had seen it before but I think even she was thrilled that we were already back and getting close to the start of our first voyage together across the Atlantic to England.

We had about a week before we sailed so we explored New Jersey and New York. We had a weekend in New York and arrived there on a Sunday, having booked into a hotel in Newark. I went downtown in New York and sold the car, I thought. The man to whom I sold it said he would give me $50 and send it to me. The day we were leaving I dumped the luggage at the pier, drove the car around to the establishment of 'Myer the Buyer' and put the key through the mail box. When I first went in to sell the car he came out to look at it and he brought one of his workers and said, 'Look what this guy drove from Nevada.' They all laughed, clapped me on the back and said I was a brave man. Having put the keys through the mailbox and forgotten that I had left my good English shoes in the car, I headed back to the ship. Naturally, I never heard from Myer the Buyer again, and as I had left the car outside his place on a deserted street it might not have been there when he opened up.

The *Queen Mary* was magnificent. We were travelling cabin class. I had never been on a liner before but Betty was quite used to the procedures and, being a seasoned traveller, she had no problem whatsoever finding the cabin and getting us stowed away, tipping porters and finding the right people to help us.

It was expensive but I never regretted it. It was a wonderful trip and five of the best days of my life. It was a great way to spend a honeymoon. I had flown into New York over the Statue of Liberty and now we were sailing past at sea level. This is one of the greatest thrills one can have, to see the Statue of Liberty from a ship.

We had no plans except to get back to the Isle of Wight and look for a job somewhere. Without the ECFMG examination I couldn't get a job anywhere in America. In spite of my long stay in Nevada I was still not completely won over to the American way of life, but of course I had not seen it at its best, living in a boarding house and working in the laundry room in the basement of a hotel! I was not determined to come back but when I arrived in England my values would be different.

Betty and I had made arrangements to have a car delivered in London. Cars were difficult to get for the British but we had applied for this from America and we got a de luxe Morris Mini. They had just come on the market and were revolutionary: front-wheel drive and simplification, and smaller than any car that had ever been produced but nevertheless roomier inside than some larger cars. We got every luxury we could get, including a roof-rack, which paid off later.

The ship was tremendous. I remember staying on deck watching New York fade in the distance. The skyscrapers, the Empire State Building, the Statue of Liberty, the energy of America one could not forget. The attention and the services on the ship were beyond anything I could have expected. Again it was not new to Betty but my open-mouthed amazement continued. The bars, dining rooms, ballrooms and the endless decks, cinemas – everything was geared to make this a floating city, which was indeed the case. I loved every minute of it, including the parties, bingo games and entertainment, right into the night. The meals were stupendous and seemingly endless. I gained 5 pounds in the 5 days it took to cross the Atlantic. We made lots of friends, exchanging addresses, hardly believing that we would never see or hear from any of them again.

We arrived at Le Havre early in the morning of the fifth day and then crossed the Channel to Southampton. The transition to the boat train to London was smooth and well organized. I was relieved to be back in England, where everything seemed to be as I expected it to be with no surprises; but I just still had the shadow of some regrets about the possibility that I might never again see the United States. Unknown to myself, I had already fallen in love with America, and one thing was sure: I would never, never forget it. I would never again think or feel as I had thought and felt before I crossed the Atlantic for the first time. It would take a while for my mixed feelings to sort themselves out but sort themselves they would.

By the time we got to London on the boat train we had regained our land legs and we headed straight for the Cumberland Hotel, this time to a single room. Our trip from Reno had been an adventure and it was wonderful doing everything with Betty as a married couple. I felt that this was the first time I was really in love with anyone. Betty's sense of humour and her worldliness and ability to handle all situations bore out how valuable she must have been to the people with whom she had worked. I was still a country boy and had a lot to learn. America would not have been as educational to me without Betty to instruct, advise and encourage me.

The following morning we picked up our new cream Mini in London, much to the envy of the staff and even the salesman who delivered it to us. They were very helpful, covering road taxation, insurance and everything when we told them we would be living for some months in England and in the Isle of Wight. All arrangements for service and upkeep of the car were made from London. We left the dealership, and the salesman was watching the car until we went around the corner at the end of the street. Back at the Cumberland we packed the car with everything we had. It was a tighter squeeze than the old Chevy in America but we got it all in. We headed straight for Southampton, stopping in a few pubs along the way to enjoy some really good English beer and a few Guinnesses.

We spent one night in Southampton and our new cream Mini was the cause of much admiration to many passers-by because new cars were so scarce in England. The next morning we caught the ferry to the island, spending the trip in the bar. When we arrived at Freshfield, we were warmly welcomed by Betty's parents. It had been a long absence but the island looked lovely even in the late autumn and our little car looked at home in the driveway at Freshfield.

We got back into the circuit of pub crawling and meeting old friends for Betty and renewing new ones for me. We had many adventures to relate to Betty's parents about our months in America.

The weather was getting cold and the skies were grey. I had no job and no prospects but I knew that as soon as I tried, everything would be fine and I'd get a job somewhere.

We met Betty's old friend Lofty in the club several mornings a week and listened to his jokes. We told him some of ours and discussed our future. He wanted us to go to South Africa, where he had intended once to go, saying that the future was now there. As a result of his heckling we decided to look into the South African situation and obtained details of how we should go about emigrating there. At the same time we also got information about Australia and New Zealand. I began perusing the advertisements for positions overseas in the *British Medical Journal*.

I wrote to my parents and told them my plans but the idea of Australia horrified my father. He said I would never see him again if I went that far. He was not as adventuresome as I, anyway. When I told him I was thinking of South Africa also, he came up with objections because of the possibility of getting a tropical disease, for example elephantiasis. This was incurable but not fatal but horribly mutilating. Medical books showed victims wheeling their testicles around in wheelbarrows because this disease caused massive distension of the lower part of the body.

My various applications came back with information all positive and encouraging for work abroad in the Colonies and elsewhere. I began to feel that the world was my oyster but we decided to winter in the island and not rush into anything. The ECFMG was the next hurdle. I continued to search the *British Medical Journal* weekly in the job section. There were lots of overseas jobs but there were also many locums in England. I had had enough of the British National Health Service as a principal practitioner. There were lots of jobs as assistants in practices all over England but I already knew that the assistant did the dirty work.

My father had made a good point that Australia and New Zealand were so far away. My parents and Betty's parents were well up in years and we would probably never see them again if we went so far away.

Our decision to stay on in England was precipitated by winter. This was to be one of the worst winters in 40 or 50 years in England. In December the snow began to fall. We awoke one morning to find ourselves snowed in. It was then I realized what a benefit it was to have our Mini with a front-wheel drive. Deep as the snow was, it posed no problem. The car, being small, was easy to turn in the driveway in front of the house. It was a good experience to drive out and not find the back wheels spinning, as had been the case in snowfalls in Ireland with the rear-wheel drive.

The buses were able to continue to travel so they cleared a lot of the snow on the main roads. A neighbour who had a tractor cleared the road from the end of the driveway to the main road. We were still able to get to Newport and make our daily visits to the pub or the club and to do the shopping.

In the New Year I decided I would look for a locum lest we ran short of money. I applied for an attractive locum in Birmingham, which supplied a flat for the doctor and his wife. I was amazed to get a reply by return. The doctor advertising was a Dublin graduate. His neighbour was a doctor who had been a great friend of mine when we were students. This was the only reference he needed as Dr Kevin O'Leary had spoken very highly of me. He wanted to know how soon I could come as he was going on holiday. I prepared immediately to leave for Birmingham, and Betty and I set off three days later. The drive to Birmingham was slow. There were no motorways in those days but we got to Birmingham in one day and contacted Dr Collins. He visited us in the hotel and brought us round to meet my old friend, Dr O'Leary. The snow was everywhere and our trip had been slowed by snow and sometimes ice, but it posed no problem to the Mini.

Dr Collins installed us in the flat, which was disappointing as it was cold and sparsely furnished with old furniture. The bed was old and very uncomfortable. The tenants in the lower flat looked after the upper one and made the bed and would make breakfast if I wished. Betty spent one week, and on the first weekend I had off I drove her back to the island and went back on my own. The locum was for one month, and in spite of the bed I enjoyed it. On the last week Betty came back as she was stranded without the car.

While I was in Birmingham there was an outbreak of smallpox in the area but both Betty and I had been vaccinated. I had some very interesting evenings with Kevin O'Leary, who had once been a heavy drinker. We had drunk a lot together in Dublin as students. He had also been in my branch of the emergency army services during the summer while we were students. He had a wonderful sense of humour and we had many adventures to recall. He had been in Africa for a while and advised me strongly to give it a shot. He said there was good money to be made there, and never to take a job unless they supplied everything. He gave me a lot of useful information. I realized this when I eventually did go to Africa. He, however, had been in East Africa, which was vastly different from West Africa, where I was to go.

When the locum ended, Betty and I bought a very large comfortable armchair in a furniture store in Birmingham. We tied it on top of the Mini, and headed back to the island. We had promised to buy a more comfortable chair for Betty's father and this was it. Looking back on this we were lucky it did not disappear from the ferry. However, we made the trip all right. Father was delighted and bequeathed his old chair to mother. We all now had very comfortable chairs from which to view the television in the evenings.

11

Ghana, West Africa

We now got serious about answering advertisements for jobs abroad. Betty had her portable typewriter and we could send out respectable letters of application. We soon had offers. One was in Liberia and one was in Ghana and Sierra Leone. The Liberian company did not offer housing and we would be expected to bring our own cooking utensils etc. That one we turned down.

We went to a diamond-mining company in London for an interview. They received us with open arms and the job was mine. I would do six months in Ghana and six months in Sierra Leone as locum for doctors taking vacations. One of the doctors was intending to retire and we would have the option of going back and staying in Ghana. The contract would be for nine months and then three months' leave back in the United Kingdom. If I had children they would educate them anywhere in Europe or England. They would fly them out and back free for their vacations. In other words, we would have two homes, one in West Africa on the compound and one in England for our three-month vacation.

There was another offer of a position in South Africa. However, if we wished to bring any children they would have to be entered on our passports when we went for interview and be ready to travel with us.

I wrote to Marie Bradley, who was looking after the children, Gloria having gone to London to take a job with her sister there. I asked Marie to bring the children to Belfast, where they would be seen and get a medical examination, the result of which would be sent to South Africa House in London so that I could have them entered on my passport. I received no reply to several letters and I now realized that Miss Bradley was not going to be cooperative. That left South Africa out as far as making a quick decision to work there.

The diamond-mining company in Ghana and Sierra Leone was now the most attractive. They paid the highest salary, covering everything. This included National Health insurance in Great Britain, all types of life insurance, bonuses for various things etc.

Betty and I decided this was worth investigating. We went again to London, where first we were interviewed by the Firestone Rubber Company. Firestone were anxious to employ me but I stalled and decided the CAST Diamond Mining Company was the most impressive. It was encouraging to know that I was in demand and I was not going to be out in the street.

I think that this experience had a lasting effect on me for the rest of my working career. Coming out of Ireland and Northern Ireland, I did not know what was waiting for me in the big world outside. I now realized that as a doctor I obviously would never have trouble getting a job. Since then I have never panicked when I found myself unemployed.

CAST was the choice and we set a date and time when we would be ready to go to Africa. That gave them time to notify the doctor I was going to replace in order that he could make his arrangements.

When we got back to the island we then had to get rid of our car. It was an export model and we were afraid that we might have to pay tax on the car if we sold it in England. We had not paid any tax when we bought it. However, the local taxation office looked at all the papers and they could produce no objection to our selling it.

Fortunately, Betty had a cousin who was interested in buying a new car and who could well afford it. This was very convenient because we sold him the car and when we were ready to go he was ready to pick it up. We transferred it to his name and drove it until we caught the boat at Yarmouth and gave the keys to Fred. We did the rounds of the pubs and spread the word that we were leaving. Goodbyes came from all and sundry but we told them we would be back in nine months.

We spent the last night in London at the Cumberland. The

following morning we were picked up by a company car and taken to the airport and given the royal treatment on our first trip to Africa.

Leaving London, our first stop was Algiers. We were allowed off the plane for a short period. We were flying with Ghana Airways. It was really hot in Algiers and the airport was crummy and as there was no place to sit down, we walked around for a short while and then went back and got on the plane. There was not much to see on the trip as it was mostly desert until we got over Nigeria, where it was jungle until we landed in Accra, Ghana. This was to be my first locum. We were met at the airport and spent the first night at the company compound in Accra.

This was my first experience of mosquito nets, and the houseman came in and explained very carefully to us how not to leave any loophole that a mosquito might get through. It was not air-conditioned and the heat and humidity was tremendous. There were fans, however, which did cool it a little but the mosquito net offset the advantage.

The food in the guest house was very tasty and well prepared. We had soup, rice and chicken, then dessert with lots of melon and fruit.

The following morning we were picked up again by a company limo and driven to the diamond mine in Akwatia. The driver gave us a copy of the *Daily Mirror* to read. I thought it was the London *Daily Mirror* but it was the *Daily Mirror* of Ghana. All the news was local and the world news was on the back page.

The roads were well paved, two-lane only. The countryside was wooded and looked extremely civilized. Along the road we had our first experience of mammy wagons. These were lorries, with seats laid longitudinally so that the passengers, mostly women, waved at us and cheered. They seemed to be full of fun, laughter and good cheer.

Our trip took about two hours, then we arrived at the gate of what looked like a huge estate with guards. We were checked by them, all armed. The driver said something and we were passed through. He brought us immediately to the guest house, which we were to occupy until the doctor left. His wife and children had already gone. He had stayed on to indoctrinate me as to how the operation was carried out: how the patients were seen, what prescriptions were written and to introduce me to the surgeon, who was from the outside but came in every day to operate in the hospital.

The hospital was tidy, with open windows and mosquito nets around the beds. There was a consulting room, where the doctor saw the patients, and a large waiting room outside.

The compound had a golf course and was very well groomed with lawns well kept. Houses were bungalow-style and all very orderly, like a London suburb.

On our first night we had dinner with Dr Messent at his home and he had invited some other bigwigs to meet the locum. Dr Messent picked us up at the guest house and because I had just arrived he told me I need not dress for dinner. Before I left England I had been given a list of tropical clothes that were necessary and among them was a dress suit and other attire. I had purchased this in Lillywhites in London.

The dinner was served by Dr Messent's house servants. One of them was called Moru. He was very tall and barefoot but dressed in a khaki uniform. All the courses were served as in a hotel. I noted that Dr Messent treated Moru really as a servant and never thanked him for anything. Glasses were on the table and a whisky bottle. Everyone helped himself or herself – nobody waited to be asked to have a drink. The men were all in evening dress and the ladies wore long gowns.

I had noted with pleasure that Dr Messent's car was a Mercedes Benz and, although it was a diesel, I knew I was going to have good transport. Motor vehicles were diesels because of the theft of petrol. The natives would have no benefit from stealing diesel fuel because they did not have diesel vehicles.

Most of the talk that evening was about home, which was England. They plied us with questions about the latest happenings, political and otherwise, in England. They were also very interested that we had been to the United States and we were able to regale them with our adventures in Nevada.

In return they told us about procedures in the diamond mines and I was amazed by some of the tales they had to tell. The most important one was that if anyone was found climbing over the fence around the camp they were shot first and questions asked afterwards.

Several people had been arrested and returned to England for stealing or trying to steal diamonds. Any diamonds found by employees in the compound belonged to the company. Employees would be arrested if found with diamonds on their person. Diamonds found outside the compound were claimed by the company as theirs but it was difficult to prove where the diamonds came from. Anyone entering or leaving was searched to make sure that no diamonds left the compound.

There was a wide diamond-mining area outside the compound and this also belonged to the company. The diamonds were mined by surface mining. This meant that the trees were cut down and removed. Then the surface area was graded and the soils sifted and checked for diamonds. In Ghana most of the diamonds were industrial and, though valuable, were not nearly as valuable as gem diamonds, which were mostly found in Sierra Leone.

When the gravel had been sifted for valuable stones, they ended up with mostly diamonds and quartz. The final check for diamonds was placing the stones or gravel on long conveyor belts on which there was a sticky substance, and to this only diamonds would adhere. The conveyor belt carried the gravel up to a point where it turned over to go under again in an ever continuous belt. As it turned over at the top, the stones of no value fell off and the diamonds stuck.

These were brought down to a lower level on another conveyor belt. This belt, however, was surrounded by glass, and through the glass there were holes. These holes were attached to gloves. The person who was going to pick the diamonds off the belt put his or her hand into the glove and dropped them off to the side. They could not ever touch the diamond except through the glove. Nobody could ever slip a diamond into his pocket or clothing and take it home.

When the diamonds were finally proven to be diamonds, they were stored in metal milk cans, which were then welded shut. These were only opened and used as the market demanded. There were dozens of these cans full of diamonds and it is said if they were all opened and put on the market diamonds would be a dime a dozen. By keeping them sealed and not allowing diamonds on the market except at a controlled rate, the value was kept up.

Diamonds are unique in that an experienced diamond dealer can know immediately from what part of Africa, even what part of the earth, they came.

A story was told of an Irishman who was hired as a guard in Ghana and got himself a bag of diamonds in various ways, nobody knows how. He arrived back in London, decided to sell his diamonds and went into a diamond store. The man behind the counter looked at them and knew that they had come from Ghana. He did not tell the Irishman, only asked where he had got them. The Irishman said he got them from South Africa and he wanted to sell them. The man told him to come back in the afternoon as the man who was the dealer was not there. The Irishman went back in the afternoon and was arrested. There was no doubt these diamonds had come from Ghana and they had been stolen. He was sent back to Ghana to be tried. This brings out the point that if diamonds are stolen they are almost impossible to dispose of.

Dr Messent stayed on for about two days to show me around and introduce me to the staff, other expatriates and the hospital staff. I met the surgeon, who was a German. He worked in a hospital run by nuns outside the compound. He came in each day, on call, to do surgery and cover whenever the doctor was away. He was a member of the CAST Club, to which Dr Messent introduced me. One was expected to go to the club each evening and socialize.

At the club there was a swimming pool and there were tennis courts and the golf course. Nobody could get bored and feel they had nothing to do while there. We made some good friends with whom we have stayed in touch until this day.

There were outlying clinics to which I went during the week. There was a chemist who filled the prescriptions in the company pharmacy. We had stores in the compound selling everything. There was a cinema, which showed movies on Sunday nights. It was going to one of these movies that I discovered that the front passenger door on the Mercedes was not 100 per cent effective.

We did not have seat belts in those days. One evening, swinging through a turn in the jungle on the way to the cinema, the door opened and Betty fell out. I did not discover this until I had already parked. This was a standing joke throughout our time in Akwatia.

Life was very social and there were receptions and parties almost every night. Each evening there was activity in the club, mostly boozing, but some dancing. On Sunday mornings there was a buffet in the club and we ate our brunch around the pool. When Dr Messent left I was in complete charge and the existence was very pleasant indeed. If any of the expatriates were ill I did house calls. They did not come to the hospital with the natives. House calls were a social event and one was expected to sit down and have a drink and a chat after the patient had been attended to.

On weekends we could go down to the beach at Winnebah near Accra and swim in the sea. There were surfboards, which it would not have been too difficult to learn to use. We could also shop in Accra on Saturdays when the diamond mines closed. Having the use of the diesel Mercedes, I was very popular. People were always hoping to be invited to Accra on Saturdays. On these trips I found the diesel to be very sluggish. When we passed the mammy wagons on the straight road they would cheer and wave. Then on the long dragging hills the diesel would slow down. The mammy wagons, which were driven by petrol, would then whizz past us and the occupants would then cheer and shout their derision as they left us far behind.

Dr Messent's three months' vacation came to an end and we were making preparations to move along the coast to Sierra Leone. I had to make a decision then if I would be interested in working permanently in Ghana or not. However, I found the disquieting news that unless I resigned from the company I could only take out half my earned salary to be a very deciding factor. I had not been told about this rule, recently brought in by President Nkrumah. This would have definitely soured the carrot which got me to Ghana in the first place. Now I began to think that maybe Firestone might have been a better choice.

The medical experience had been enormous and new in Ghana. I saw diseases that I had never seen previously. Yaws had been a terrible disease in the past, causing deep ulcers and wide rotting ulcers of the feet. Penicillin now cured it and the ulcers cleared up completely. When I saw them first I could not imagine that they would ever get better. Malaria was rampant and we took anti-malarial medication all the time we were there. I escaped infection although Betty did come down with a bout towards the end of our tour. Measles was deadly and ubiquitous. Children brought in with measles could get pneumonia and die overnight. It happened to several patients while I was there. This was enlightening because measles that I had seen in all my medical career in Europe was considered benign.

Sickle-cell disease was quite common and in exacerbation caused great discomfort, joint inflammation and abdominal pain, and could also be fatal. Africans had probably all suffered from malaria but it did not seem to have the severe sickening effect that it did on the Europeans. Elephantiasis I never did see.

The German surgeon was excellent and was fazed by nothing. He could not, however, do much for a patient whose arm got caught in the machinery of the separating machine which operated the continuous sticky belt. He was brought in with his arm, in a sack, having had it ripped out at the shoulder. He was not bleeding because of the shrinking of the blood vessels and flesh at the shoulder joint. He did complain bitterly when he saw his arm, from which his watch had been stolen. Plastic surgery for the remains of his shoulder was all that was needed. He never showed any signs of shock or other problems.

Children who were in the hospital were brought presents by their families, who stayed in the hospital with them and cooked and looked after them. They had a custom of bringing the child a bird tied on a string so that the bird flew around the bed with the string tied to its leg. I made a fuss about this when I went there first but I was advised to back off as this had been going on for years. It was best left alone and I should just ignore it.

My experience in Ghana left me well prepared for Sierra Leone. Dr Messent arrived back one day and I left the next.

12

Sierra Leone, West Africa

The flight from Accra, Ghana to Freetown, Sierra Leone, took about two hours in the propeller plane, flying over the top of the Ivory Coast and Liberia to get there.

The airport in Freetown was much smaller and less organized than the one in Accra but it was quite efficient. We were met by a company limo and brought to a very comfortable guest house. The food, as in Ghana, was very palatable and well prepared. While there we had the use of a car and driver. We had to wait until a plane came from Tongo, which was the compound at which I was to spend the next six months.

The following morning we got a chance to go out to a beach and it was the most wonderful beach I ever saw. There was nobody on it but us. It stretched as far as the eye could see and the water was warm and calm. We were supplied with a delicious picnic basket for lunch and we swam and lay in the sun until we were picked up in the afternoon and brought back to Freetown.

That evening we met the pilot, Ted Nutt, who was to fly us to Tongo the following day. The company plane was a Beaver and Ted was very particular. We had to sit exactly where he told us to sit and put our bags exactly where he wanted them to be put. Apparently this was to keep the plane in balance. I had never been in such a small plane and we flew quite low and close to the treetops of the jungle. It was a very interesting flight.

There was a big airfield at Tongo and when we touched down we were met by Nonie Cook, who was the manageress of the camp. Her husband, George, was an engineer with the company.

At the airport there was an almost new Volkswagen waiting for me and this was to be our transport while we were in Sierra Leone. It was like having an old friend. I had had two Volkswagens in Ireland before I left, one of which was involved in the fatal accident which caused me finally to leave.

Nonie brought us to the guest house, where we spent the first night. Our food was brought in and it was like a mini-hotel with the usual mosquito precautions. However, this bedroom was air-conditioned.

After breakfast the following morning, we moved into the doctor's residence, where there was also an air-conditioned bedroom. The doors and windows were screened throughout the house and there were ample fans. We had two houseboys, who did not speak good English and were not nearly as polished as Moru, whom we had left in Ghana. The comparison with Moru all during the time we were in Sierra Leone made us sad every time we remembered him. The servants here were surly, unresponsive and probably stupid. By and large we found the people to be much less friendly than the Ghanaians.

When we had been in Ghana we had not really appreciated it because it was the first African community we had ever been in. We remembered the fact that the Ghanaian women are famous for their beauty and their ability to dance and sing. Comparing all this with Sierra Leone, we now saw the difference.

Many of the Sierra Leone men had filed their teeth to a sharp point, resulting in sharp jagged teeth. This, I was told, indicated that they were cannibals.

One morning the Chief of Police of the camp asked me to identify some bones in the barracks. I identified a crushed skull and some clean white bones and confirmed that the skull had been smashed by a blunt object and was not the result of the victim having fallen from a tall palm tree. I was friendly with a wine seller who collected wine from palm trees by climbing them, using a hoop around his shoulders and shinning up like a squirrel. He had been missing for some time and probably had been killed and eaten by cannibals and the bones placed at the foot of a tree with his hoop.

The Scottish Chief of Police had arrested some suspects and

asked me to stay and see him use his lie detector. There was a large patch of white sand in front of the police barracks and there the suspects were placed in a line-up. The policeman then stood in front of them, telling them he would find the guilty one and have him hanged.

The policeman told me that the guilty parties would sweat with fear and the sand under their feet would darken. I believed it when I saw that only three perspired under their feet.

I left Sierra Leone before their trial in Freetown so I did not hear the outcome.

When we had problems with the servants we sent for Nonie Cook, who lived about 100 yards away. She could speak their language and they were all afraid of her.

There had been a new hospital built and it was very elaborate, with modern beds, modern kitchen and an up-to-date operating room. The surroundings were beautiful. The old hospital was still being used as an outpatient dispensary. It was open to the elements and there was about a foot separation between the roof and the walls. This kept it aerated and there was always a breeze. I needed an interpreter to speak to the patients because none of them spoke English. My interpreter was also the chemist, a surly, antagonistic gentleman who wore very thick glasses. I had my doubts from the beginning if his interpreting was accurate or not. He apparently considered himself a doctor and did not think there was any need for my presence in the hospital at all. On a few occasions when I went back in the afternoon after the clinic had closed, I found him treating patients.

The club was very nicely laid out and there was a swimming pool and tennis court. It was not in the same class as the club in Ghana but, being smaller, it was more like an English pub. Everyone spoke to everyone else. In the large club in Ghana people grouped themselves and kept to their own tables. In fact, it lent itself to cliques. Tongo was different. Everybody greeted everybody else. We all knew everyone by their first names and it was a much more friendly club, and camp.

Nonie Cook kept the whole thing going and arranged curry parties and buffets etc. There was never a dull moment when she was around. Her husband, George, was very droll and humorous.

We were fortunate to have them living next door to us and had many visits back and forth during our stay.

The main camp and head office for Sierra Leone was in Yengema, which was about 75 miles away. The road was mountainous and unsurfaced. It could be reached in a short trip by plane if the necessity arose. Ted Nutt flew back and forth regularly between Yengema, Tongo and Freetown. He also brought the mail in every day to Tongo.

We had no outlying clinics in Sierra Leone, as there were in Ghana, and the doctor in Yengema was also a surgeon. He could fly down to Tongo to perform surgery if anything came up that could not be transferred to Yengema.

The same rules applied as far as taking diamonds in or out of the compound. However, the diamonds in Sierra Leone were gem diamonds and much more valuable. As in Ghana, the compound was well secured.

The clinic only opened in the morning so I had the afternoons free. Every afternoon there was a storm with heavy rain and we could get fresh water off the roof; it was very soft. Betty on several occasions stood under the roof and washed her hair.

The afternoons being free, I decided to dictate a synopsis of *Beaumont's Medical Textbook* to Betty, and as she could type so fast she could type it directly, headings and all. I figured that if I did that before I left Africa, studying for the ECFMG examination would be relatively easy, at least for the medical part.

My calculations were wide of the mark. I finally found that the only way to study for this examination was to get multiple-choice examination books. These were not available until I got back to mainland America, so my hard work on the synopsis of *Beaumont* was in vain. Betty at least learned a lot about medicine!

Every week we made a trip to a small town called Kenema. There we could obtain food that was not available in the camp and there was a local post office. The camp store occasionally got large 5-gallon containers of good Portuguese wine, wrapped in plaster of Paris and surrounded by basket weave. We could also get British beer, Scotch whisky and gin, so our parties could be made very enjoyable.

The club was open from about four in the afternoon until nine in the evening. There was a lot of entertainment because there were always a few characters there who could be depended upon to produce a few laughs. There was piped music, record players and some dancing. Every so often Nonie would organize a party, a play or an evening's entertainment.

Nonie and George had a dog, a wire-haired terrier called Corky. He was untouchable and many people got bitten trying to pat him on the head. He also had strong sexual prowess and there was rarely a day but he had become entangled with some female dog from the compound, usually outside our window. The Cooks went on leave before we left and the camp was dull without them. Later we met them in England when we went home.

The night before we left we had a party at the club and we were given a royal send-off. Dr Jaques, the permanent doctor in the camp, returned the following morning on the plane on which we left for Freetown. We went home via the Canary Islands and spent a few days there. The Hotel Santa Catalina in Las Palmas was magnificent as was the food. We toured the island and the weather was perfect.

We left the sun behind and arrived in England in a fog. We had rented a car, which picked us up at the railway station in Southampton, where we arrived in pouring rain. After spending the night in Southampton at the Polygon Hotel we left the following morning for the island.

As usual we were very welcome and we had a joyous reunion with Betty's parents.

Soon we were back to our pub crawls and meetings with Lofty in a new pub that he had discovered called The Falcon. It was run by a great character called Fred Attrill, with whom we became very friendly. We never missed a morning in his jolly pub with a bunch of workmen, Lofty and lunchtimers.

Now that I had the time I decided to make a good effort to obtain my children again. I requested to have them brought to be medically examined for South Africa or the United States because they would have to immigrate, as I had.

Within two weeks I was served papers that Marie Bradley was making my children wards of court in her custody. Gloria was apparently still working in England so she was certainly not with the children, who were still with Marie Bradley.

I went to my solicitor in the Isle of Wight and when he saw the situation he told me it would be a long and hard battle. I would have to go to Northern Ireland to testify, get a solicitor over there, then go into court and contend with any lawyers Gloria or her sister had got into the act. The whole thing was going to become more complicated and would slow up any plans I had for going to South Africa or returning to America. I had thought of going to Canada with the children but that was now prevented.

All I could do was to sign the papers and send them back. If I wanted to contest the decision at any time I would have to go back to Northern Ireland. My solicitor told me it was not going to be worth it. There was always the possibility that they would appeal Gloria's divorce and look for a greater amount of support than she was getting. I agreed to pay the children's support to Marie Bradley and continue to pay it until they were 18 years of age.

My parents were also paying Marie Bradley an additional 25 per cent of what I had been paying, so she was well looked after.

She had the nerve to write to me later, asking me if I could help her to pay her lawyer's bill as she had incurred quite a bit of expense in making the children wards of court! That, of course, did not deserve a reply and I presumed that much of the children's money was going to that cause anyway.

The winter was long so I did locums in England and in various parts of the country as well as the Isle of Wight. I began to answer advertisements in the *Medical Journal* for positions in the United States. I had finally decided that the United States was the only direction in which I should go if I was going to succeed and become independent of my previous problems.

The children could have free education in Northern Ireland. Gloria would eventually return there and would get unemployment benefit and free medical treatment. The children would also have free medical treatment and Marie Bradley could collect family allowances and various other benefits. It so happened that the children got scholarships because of the fact that they had no access to their parents. The blame for difficulties was always placed on me and not on Marie Bradley, who had really instigated the whole disaster.

As far as I know, Gloria stayed away from the children and never went near them. They did visit her in Belfast, until she died suddenly there in 1975.

I continued to study between locums and the island and tried again for the examination in London in March, although I was poorly prepared. Naturally, I didn't pass. I kept applying for positions in the United States. Some were attractive and some not, but I finally was offered a nice position as an extern in Norwalk, Connecticut.

13

United States and Canada

We prepared again and were ready to travel at the end of June 1963 on the *United States*. While we were travelling westwards, President Kennedy was travelling eastwards and touring Ireland.

When we arrived in Norwalk I was given a free apartment and Betty got a job as the secretary in the Tumour Clinic at Norwalk Hospital. I was working as an extern in anticipation of my passing the ECFMG exam in September. If I passed, I was promised an internship at the hospital. It was pleasant and I had plenty of time to study in the library, which had all the latest medical books and the question-and-answer books I needed. It was the first time I had seen the books which I needed to study for the examination.

However, in September when I sat the exam I didn't make the 75 per cent necessary, so we decided to look at the Canadian situation. There were lots of jobs advertised in the *Canadian Medical Journal* which were paying well. One which seemed appropriate was in Virgil, Ontario, almost next door to Niagara on the Lake. I telephoned the doctor there and he employed me at my own figure.

We had bought an old Ford, about six years old, so we packed once more and headed for Canada. My green card was still current. When I reached the border the Canadians were not interested in it but just asked me where I was going. I told them and they said I would have to immigrate if I was going to work. The paperwork was done in an hour, our passports stamped and we entered Canada.

The doctor was a Ukranian and he ran a large practice, much of it surgical. He had a large European clientele because he could speak every language in Europe. There was a German doctor who came in and gave anaesthetics and he told me he would teach me how to do it. In a week I was giving anaesthetics, doing general practice, family practice, obstetrics and gynaecology. It was like being back in Ireland because it was a rural community and much of the practice was house calls.

Many of the patients were children for tonsillectomies, of which the doctor did three or four every morning and I gave the anaesthetics.

We rented a house which had a large furnace in the middle of the small kitchen. This was the only heating but it did heat the water. The whole inside of the house was overgrown with potted vines and plants. We tidied the whole thing up and removed the plants, which left a lot more space and a cleaner house. However, when the owners paid a visit and found the plants were gone there was quite a storm. I thought they would never get over it. They may never have! Looking back, it must have taken them years to grow all that. Plants were growing through from the kitchen into the living room from roots in pots beside the furnace. It was an indoor jungle.

At this time there was heavy snow and I had to be ploughed out every morning to be able to get to the hospital. When I came home the snow was piled along the street and across the driveway, so I couldn't get in again. Sometimes I had to park on the street. If I got a night call this posed quite a problem. Keeping the driveway clear before the snow froze was almost impossible.

At this time President Kennedy was assassinated, which left us all very sad indeed. What made us more sad was that my boss was delighted that President Kennedy was killed because he said the President was going soft on Communism.

Betty decided it would be best for her to visit England and spend Christmas with her parents. We had visited some of her friends in Eastern Ontario, namesakes of hers but not relatives, and they had invited me for Christmas. The clinic would be closed over the holiday and this gave me the chance to visit the Ontario Jackmans.

My Ford was giving me a lot of problems so I brought it into a garage in St Catherines, where they had a nice Volkswagen for sale. Volkswagens were not popular yet but I knew them from way back. I quickly made a deal, trading my Ford for the Volkswagen, which I knew would be serviceable. It also had a roof-rack, which would prove very helpful. It behaved well in snow, having all the weight over the back wheels. It was almost as good as the Mini.

I had a very enjoyable Christmas with the Jackmans and had an uneventful trip back again to Virgil.

Just after the New Year the doctor presented me with several books of receipts for anaesthetics, and I began to sign them as he asked me – they had already been filled in. However, I began to notice that I could not possibly have given as many anaesthetics as I was signing receipts for. I asked to see the medical records. He told me that I did not need to do that, and so did his secretary – just sign the receipts and send them in. I thought otherwise and confronted the doctor, who looked quite guilty. I went home, and after I had counted the number of signatures needed in the book, there was no possibility that I could have given that many anaesthetics. I called him on the phone and I heard his wife in the background say, 'Fire him.'

I immediately got my *Medical Journal* out again and began looking for another job. I found a nice advertisement for a position in the Queen Elizabeth Hospital in Toronto. The salary was not nearly as much as I was making in Virgil but it sounded very attractive. There was a phone number and I called. When I spoke to Dr Goodwin he was very interested and asked me to come to visit him. I went to see him the next day and explained my problem. He regretted that he could not pay anything like I was getting but he could supply me with sleeping accommodation in the hospital until such time as Betty came back. He told me that I could start as soon as I was available. I returned to Virgil, collected my outstanding salary and left.

Dr Goodwin, a lawyer and a physician, was a very charming and kind man. He was very tall, 6 foot 3 inches, and we were like Mutt and Jeff. He showed me over the Queen Elizabeth Hospital, which was an excellent home for the elderly and those needing protracted care. It was spotless, the nursing was of the best and there were no examples of neglect or bedsores. Patients were got out of bed every day. The floors were scrubbed and in the corridors and wards there was a general smell of cleanliness. The grounds were beautifully kept and there was a lovely roof terrace. The patients were brought up there every day if they were capable of going up to sit in the sun and enjoy the view over Toronto. It was a wonderful place to work and I had the company of another doctor who was working full-time. Dr Zeffers was a Lithuanian and a very kind and thoughtful man.

There was a South African doctor who was in private practice in Toronto and he visited every morning of the week. He was a great help showing me the ropes and was extremely amusing and a very able physician. He also did some surgery when the need arose.

Not all the patients were indigent and some paid privately. By and large the home for the elderly was as well run – if not the best run – as any I have ever been in before or since.

I was given a very nice little room situated in the nurses' quarters. There was a beautiful large sitting room around it and a grand piano which I could play in the evenings if I wished. I also had a radio in my room. The heating was perfect but could get too hot if I did not watch the radiators.

Dr Goodwin made me his assistant and told me he would pay me more, except that I had been getting paid more than he was. I was treated very generously indeed.

Betty was having a lot of worries with my moving around but I kept her in touch and at the end of January she returned from England. With her expected return I obtained an apartment in a high-rise not far from the hospital. The lady in charge was very kind and did everything to make the apartment comfortable. It was a one-bedroom furnished apartment facing out onto a narrow alley. Echoes could be heard when the windows were open but the price was right and there was an elevator.

We occasionally went across to Buffalo, New York, on weekends, and although we were rarely stopped, one American Customs man asked to see our identification. When he saw our green cards he said that these would have to be registered in the New Year to maintain our immigration status. We were advised to bring them along with our passports the next time we were going through. When we did we found that this was a fatal mistake. We later discovered that we could have come in and out without registering.

Anyway, we did, and when they saw from our passports that we had been stamped in as Canadian citizens they confiscated our green cards and sent us back into Canada. From then on we had to carry our passports with us and that was our exit and entry permit to the United States. We were told that we could appeal the confiscation but that our case would have to be heard and we would have to give good cause for returning to the United States. This started long correspondence back and forth with the Immigration authorities in Buffalo, to no apparent end.

However, I sat for the ECFMG examination in March 1964 and passed. This put a completely different complexion on the immigration status. I could now explain that I left the United States because I had not passed the examination. I could now take a job in the United States. This was entirely feasible and we were called in front of a judge in Buffalo, New York, at the border post. We had a hearing and he granted the return of our green cards. He stipulated that we should enter the United States as soon as possible and have our passports corrected, deleting the Canadian citizenship.

It was the greatest relief that we could return to the United States. I began immediately getting copies of the *American Medical Association Journal* and looking for jobs and agencies. I had an offer of a residency in psychiatry in the United States and I went for interviews at various hospitals in New York and Michigan. These were within driving distance.

When I saw the mental institution in Buffalo it reminded me of the Dark Ages, with patients up on various floors in cages shouting down to their relatives.

I decided then to go into Michigan and look at a mental hospital there where they had a residential programme. Betty and I were shown through many locked doors with security everywhere. We were interviewed by a lady doctor with an Eastern European accent who was wearing her wig backwards. She showed us around the hospital and we looked through the windows of padded cells at patients who were stark naked, being fed under the doors like animals. This convinced me that psychiatry was not my idea of a medical career. I knew I just couldn't hack it.

The next offer I got was in Roxbury, Boston, in the Jewish Memorial Hospital. It was a minimum wage but I figured I could live on it. The position in Toronto was made more palatable by the fact that Betty worked in the Massey Ferguson offices as a secretary. She was making more money than I was at the hospital. We now decided that she could also get a job in Boston and we could survive until such time as I got a residency.

We went to Boston and I was interviewed by the administrator of the hospital. He painted a glowing picture and introduced us to other doctors on the staff. They were all pleasant and I decided to take this position. We returned to Toronto and told Dr Goodwin of our good news, which he told us was his bad news. He advised us strongly to go for the career angle and make hay while we were still young.

Dr Goodwin and our landlady were the only friends we had in Toronto and we said goodbye and headed for Boston in our Volkswagen, which was packed to the roof, plus the roof-rack. We stopped off in Albany, New York, to spend a few days in the sun. The motel was a Schrafts with a beautiful pool. Spending so much time in the pool absolutely fried us. We both got badly sunburned and had to extend our stay. Finally, we got on the road again and made good time. I found that getting in the lee of large trucks was the only way we could make a speed over 55 m.p.h. in our loaded Volkswagen. Getting behind the trucks, we could make as much time as they did. I learned from truck drivers later that it was a terror when anyone did that. If they slowed down suddenly, the car behind would not be able to stop in time. Our time was not yet up so we made it.

We got into Boston in the middle of the night, with no map and no idea where we were going. Eventually, we ended up in a very nice motel in Beacon Street.

It was very hot in Boston and the weather we had experienced in Albany lasted all during the trip. The car was not air-conditioned and even in the middle of the night in Boston while we were looking for a hotel the heat was stifling.

It was after midnight when we found the Beacon Street Motel. Because we were guests, the night porter opened the bar and we had some beer. That was the coldest and most welcome beer I can ever remember drinking.

The following day we got a map of the city and oriented ourselves, and after a hearty breakfast set out for the Jewish Memorial Hospital. Boston was a very impressive and beautiful city. We eventually found a way to Roxbury and to the hospital.

It was situated in very pleasant grounds but obviously had been built piecemeal. Finding one's way around was difficult at first. The Administrator was very nice and gave me a great welcome. He told me I could start as soon as I wished. He introduced me to the Chief of Staff, a very pleasant Egyptian gentleman who was very well educated medically. He really ran the whole hospital when the attending staff had left.

Betty and I then went to search for an apartment, preferably furnished. We eventually found one on Cleveland Circle in Brookline. When we were settled in, I started work at the Jewish Memorial. The staff were very nice to work with. The nurses were very obliging and helpful and the patients were mostly elderly.

The standard of nursing was very high, and although there were some chronic patients and no emergency room type of medicine, it was really run as a hospital.

There was a full-time laboratory, X-ray Department and Rehabilitation and Physical Medicine Department. On the whole, it was a much more active type of hospital than the Queen Elizabeth had been. Visiting staff came every day and did rounds. They admitted and discharged patients and were always available for consultation. During the night, whoever was on night duty – which I was on every fifth night – consulting staff were always available by phone. They were ready to come in on emergencies. The beds were divided and each doctor had so many patients to visit at least once daily. The doctor visited them again when the patient's personal physician visited the hospital. The visiting physicians were all first-class and board certified. They treated the house physicians as equals and frequently had lunch with us in the cafeteria. There was a comfortable dormitory for night-duty physicians and on the whole the job was not difficult. All lab facilities were available around the clock.

Betty decided that she would like to try for a job in the city. On one of her first applications she succeeded in obtaining a job with an attorney who had been a senator in the past. He still called himself Senator. His name was not Kennedy. Betty could travel to work on the streetcar, which let her off two or three blocks from her office. Financially, we were as well off as we had been in Toronto.

The Boston Strangler was on the loose during our stay in Boston. This did not leave Betty feeling too secure on the nights that I spent in the hospital. However, the building in which our apartment was, was fairly well secured and the windows looked inwards onto a courtyard. We were on the third floor. Access was not as ready as it was in some of the apartments and houses where the Strangler had visited. Our building was built specifically as an apartment building and was not an adapted family or boarding house, as some of the Strangler's haunts turned out to be.

The hospital Chief of Staff had had to leave Egypt because he was Jewish. He was a very jolly and friendly gentleman with whom I stayed in touch many years after I left. There was a German–Spanish doctor on the staff who had been ambassador to a South American country, but when his ambassadorship ended he had decided to immigrate to the United States. He and his wife were very friendly.

My brother Cairbre, also a doctor, was at this time running a rehabilitation centre in New Hampshire, called Crotched Mountain Foundation. When I was established I called him one evening. He was very glad to hear from me and decided that he would come down to Boston to visit. He spent an evening with us and we had dinner and drinks. He came up with the suggestion that I should get into rehabilitation medicine as I had had the experience in Toronto and was now connected with rehabilitation programmes in the Jewish Hospital.

I decided to think it over. After about a week I contacted him again and he suggested that I take a few days off and we all go to New York and visit Dr Rusk.

Cairbre had been in Newfoundland when there was an outbreak of polio and he became very interested in rehabilitation, especially of post-poliomyelitis patients. As a result of his experience he applied for a residency with the New York University at the Rusk Institute run by Dr Howard Rusk. When he completed his residency there, he got the job as Administrator and Chief in the Crotched Mountain Foundation in Greenfield, New Hampshire. By now he was well established and a well-recognized physiatrist. He knew everyone and everything that was to be known about the relatively new specialty of Physical Medicine and Rehabilitation.

He picked us up in Boston one morning in the summer of 1964. He drove us to New York, where we had an appointment to meet Dr Howard Rusk to discuss the possibility of me coming to do a residency where Cairbre had been.

On the way down, Cairbre suggested that we call to see Dr Robcliff Jones at Yale University. Dr Jones had a vacancy for a resident in physical medicine and rehabilitation. While we were with Dr Jones he mentioned that he knew another Irishman who had been with him at the Mayo Clinic in Rochester when he did his residency, a man called Dr Walter Treanor, better known as Wally Treanor.

This was a magnificent coincidence because Wally had been in the same year as I was in the University College, Dublin. We had been close friends and I had been his secretary when he was Auditor of the UCD Literary and Historical Society, a world-famed debating society in the university. When I was an intern Wally was the Chief Resident in St Vincent's Hospital, Dublin. We had got to know each other very well but we had lost touch completely. I had known he was in the United States but not where. Now Rob Jones was able to tell me all about him and where he was and how to get in touch with him. The fact that I was so friendly with Wally changed his whole attitude, but he said he could not pay me very much if I got the residency.

We said goodbye and went on to New York to see Dr Rusk, who was also very helpful. He could come up with four times as much as Rob Jones was aware of and he gave me all the papers and information necessary to get grants and to have a reasonable salary while going through a residency there. We spent the night in New York and hotfooted it back to Rob Jones when we were going through New Haven. It was a Saturday morning but he obliged by coming in to meet us again. When Cairbre told him about the finances that Howard Rusk had available, Rob said, 'Well, if Howard can do it, so can I.' He told me to wait for him and he would investigate getting me more money if I went to Yale. Meanwhile, he gave me all the forms and information for me to be a resident at Yale University.

On the way back we were filled with glee and the prospects looked very good indeed. I spoke to some of the visiting physicians at the Jewish Memorial Hospital and told them I would probably be making an application for Yale. Of course they said that being a foreigner I wouldn't get in, but they would certainly write me good references nevertheless.

I then wrote to Toronto to Dr Goodwin and to a doctor who was a patient in the Queen Elizabeth Hospital. He was an internationally famous geneticist. By return mail I got glowing references from all the people from whom I had requested them.

Next I got a telephone call from Rob Jones telling me that he could get me an $11,000 annual grant, which was the maximum that Dr Rusk could get me. I returned to New Haven and visited him again. He told me that my references looked as though I had written them myself and there would be no difficulty in getting me appointed.

My next problem was to tell the Administrator of the hospital in Boston, who had been so nice to me when I arrived. I told him that I was taking a residency at Yale starting 1 January 1965. He was furious and became rude and threatening. He told me that if I left he would sue me because I had a contract for a year and had only done half of it. The rest of our contact was by mail when I tendered my resignation, collected my last salary and left.

Later, when I applied for United States citizenship, this same Administrator refused to give me a letter verifying that I had spent six months in Boston. His secretary obliged anyway, without telling her boss what she had done.

* * *

I had nowhere to stay in New Haven when I left Boston, so we decided that Betty should go again to England and spend Christmas with her parents. Cairbre invited me to spend Christmas with them in Crotched Mountain. We gave notice in our apartment and saw Betty off by plane from Logan airport. It was a full moon that night and an eclipse was taking place. I had the car packed with everything we had and I followed Cairbre and Ethna up to Crotched Mountain.

Christmas in Crotched Mountain was really enjoyable. I didn't bother to unload the car. It was tightly packed with equipment on top as well as inside and under the trunk. I left right after Christmas to get established in New Haven, Connecticut.

I had some regrets leaving Boston because I had enjoyed my stay there. I liked the hospital and the work, as well as the city itself. Betty, however, was glad to get out of it because of the Boston Strangler being still at large.

The trip to New Haven was uneventful except that some cars passing me on the thruway waved and kept pointing to my roof-rack. I figured something must be getting loose. I pulled over and found that the electric fan had blown off. I went back but never found it. It was beginning to snow and a fan would certainly not be important. I arrived in New Haven in a snowstorm but as I was now fairly well acquainted with the city, I knew my way around and checked into the YMCA.

14

Yale, New Haven

The first week in New Haven I spent looking for an apartment and being shown around Yale–New Haven Hospital, where I would spend most of my residency. Dr Jones was very kind and helpful. He established me as sharing a hospital residency with the other resident, Dr Ian MacLean. The chief resident, a lady, was sick. She had just come out of hospital so she was not present.

During the week it transpired that the lady doctor had been booked into a prosthetics course in New York University. As she could not attend, and the money had been paid, Dr Jones decided to send me down in her stead so as not to lose the spot as well as the money.

He gave me $200 in cash, told me to catch a train to New York, check into the George Washington Hotel, which was not far from the university, and attend the course for a week. I was to bring back my notes and give the department a dissertation when I returned.

Looking back on it, I was lucky to get by in a crummy hotel in a crummy part of New York carrying $200 cash around in my pocket, but I survived.

This was my first experience of tuition in America and I was very impressed. I thought it was unusual that anatomy was being taught by a non-physician. In all the universities I had been in, there were physicians teaching anatomy and nothing else. This man taught us the anatomy necessary for the fitting and teaching of patients to use prostheses (artificial limbs on their lower extremities).

The course was step by step and we were given notes, so no writing was necessary. It was an excellent course and it stood by me for the rest of my life. I never again had a problem with prostheses after this. The teaching methods and the different people who came and taught the courses were excellent. Some of them were doctors from the Rusk Institute of Rehabilitation in New York. Others were staff of the university and some were professional prosthetists.

I went down to New York just about knowing what a prosthesis was and went back to New Haven an authority. I was always put in charge of the prosthetic clinic at Yale and after a few weeks I realized I knew more about prosthetics than anybody in the department. The exception was the visiting prosthesis maker who came down from Hartford. I even impressed him and he occasionally asked my advice. This gave me a great standing and a good start.

We had weekly meetings, chaired by Dr Jones, and discussed various modalities of the specialty of rehabilitation. I quickly picked up knowledge and daily I did rounds with Dr Atkins, who was a senior member of the staff. He taught me almost everything I learned in the rehabilitation residency at Yale.

There was another senior physician, who spent most of his time doing electromyography. He was very busy and rarely had time to teach. That was one of the subjects which I left New Haven being almost completely in the dark about. The doctor was an excellent lecturer and has written books on various aspects of rehabilitation. However, to take a resident or intern in hand and sit him down and teach him to do electromyography was beyond his capabilities. It took me years before I finally got the hang of this. When I did, I found it to be quite a simple procedure with no mystery in it whatsoever.

Doing rounds with Dr Atkins was fun and extremely educational. He was an erudite physician in all aspects of medicine. He had done his residency in the Rusk Institute in New York, and in Warm Springs, Georgia, with Bob Bennet.

Dr Jones was busy running the department and deeply involved with the politics and meetings related to Yale University and the hospital. He did, however, give some excellent lectures in patient examination and history taking. His notes have been useful to me during my practice of rehabilitation medicine.

Dr MacLean had the same problem I had in learning electromyography, but he went on to become one of the foremost electromyographers in the United States, if not the world. Ian left Yale at the end of his residency and went to work in Wallingford, Connecticut, with Dr Tom Hines in a very advanced rehabilitation hospital. I was promoted to Chief Resident after he left.

Shortly after this, I did a three-month stint in the rehabilitation hospital in Wallingford, known as Gaylord Hospital. Dr Tom Hines was in charge and I learned much of the practical side of rehabilitation from him and his staff.

About February 1965 Betty returned from England on the *Queen Elizabeth* and I met her in New York. We returned to the small apartment which I had rented in New Haven. It was very noisy, however, and we eventually moved to a high-rise on York Street. This was within walking distance of the hospital. We scantily furnished the apartment and found it very comfortable.

Betty decided we could not live on the resident's fellowship income and went job-hunting. She applied for a job in the Second National Bank in downtown New Haven and was employed immediately. She was personal secretary to the Vice President of the Trust Department. She enjoyed her job and made many friends there. While she was there the bank was held up during the lunch hour but she was not involved.

We lived very frugally as the apartment was quite expensive. We did get a break in June when Dr Jones and his family went on vacation to Europe. He asked us if we would house-sit for him in Fairfield and invited us out to see it. When we saw his beautiful house we jumped at the opportunity and spent six wonderful weeks that summer in absolute luxury. There was maid service and all meals were provided. Breakfast was prepared in the morning and dinner when we got back at night. We had every luxury we could wish for. We thought the long drive into work every day was worth it and we were almost sorry to see Dr Jones and his family return. Back to plain fare again.

Cairbre came to visit in the autumn and we both went to the annual Convention of Physical Medicine and Rehabilitation in

Philadelphia. The meetings of the Congress of Rehabilitation Medicine and the American Academy were held at the same time. Cairbre introduced me to many famous physiatrists and re-introduced me to Dr Rusk. I met everybody who was of any importance in my specialty.

Coming to the end of the year, it was considered that I could do rounds on my own and no longer be under the tutelage of Dr Atkins. However, we both still made a visit to the high-rise section of the hospital each morning and had coffee and muffins together. We continued this until Dr Atkins left early in 1966. With Dr McLean gone and no one else to do the work, I was the chief bottle-washer for the last year of my residency at Yale–New Haven.

Towards the end of my final year, at Christmas, I began to get ready to leave and to look for a job in rehabilitation medicine. There was very little available and I began to think of maybe going to Australia, where I heard that rehabilitation was beginning to give rise to some interest. Betty, who had been in Australia, was quite interested in investigating that further.

We decided that we would move to England and spend Christmas with Betty's parents. I did not want to go to Ireland if I could avoid it because I did not know what Marie Bradley would come up with next. We began to get ready for the trip, saying goodbye to all my friends at Yale–New Haven Hospital. I had spent some time in the Neurology, Neurosurgery and Orthopaedic Departments so I had made many friends.

There were still no positions available in rehabilitation anywhere in the United States. I was beginning to think I was up a blind alley and that this specialty had been a mistake. Little was I to know that in about ten years there would be rehabilitation jobs going begging.

Finally, December came and the certificates were given out. I received mine as Resident and Chief Resident and as a Post Doctoral Fellow. I had got the first part of the Connecticut licensing exam and had succeeded in getting a New Hampshire State licence by reciprocity. That left me an opportunity to work with the Veterans Administration if all else failed. So America was not closed to me yet.

We left our apartment in the middle of December and took a train from New Haven to New York, where we checked into the Hilton Hotel. We would have two days there before embarking on the *Queen Elizabeth* sailing for Southampton.

On the morning we were to sail we nearly panicked because we had a trunk and suitcases which the porter had piled out on the pavement outside the hotel and left. As soon as the taxi drivers saw the pile they drove away and would not stop. We gave the doorman $10, which prompted him to guarantee he would get us a taxi. He did, after about four attempts, and we were off with the luggage and heading for the docks.

Upon arrival in England, where we had pre-arranged to rent a car, we headed for the island. Again we were back into the lap of our family and had a wonderful welcome back.

Rather than prolong renting a car, I decided to buy one on the island as I could use it to do locums. I got a Ford Anglia and found it very satisfactory. It was guaranteed for as long as we had it and they promised to buy it back if we wanted to dispose of it.

Christmas was very enjoyable as we were back on our rounds and pub crawls with Lofty in the mornings and our friends in The Falcon. We had no idea at this point what we were going to do next.

I did make a trip to Ireland and visited my parents in Dublin. There was a chance of a position in Saskatchewan, Canada, where there was a doctors' strike and they were looking for doctors. I met one of the recruiters in Dublin, who was making very attractive offers. My father said, 'No! Canada is the last place you should go, especially Saskatchewan.'

When I got back to England there was still no progress until suddenly on 14 January 1967 I got a telegram from my brother in New Hampshire telling me there was a position available for a physiatrist in Louisville, Kentucky. He gave me the address and I got in touch with a Dr Smith there. Dr Smith telephoned me early in February inviting me to come to be interviewed. He volunteered my expenses from the Atlantic seaboard to Louisville.

My decision was to go back to the United States and stay with my brother in New Hampshire, using that as my base to go to

Louisville. Cairbre met me in Boston and I was able to fly from New Hampshire to Louisville for the interview.

The interview was successful and I was appointed to start working as the Associate Medical Director with Dr Smith in the middle of March 1967.

It was a beautifully equipped rehabilitation centre, having been recently renovated, and was attached to the Jewish Hospital in Louisville. It was also part of the University of Louisville.

The board of the hospital was a very busy bunch of gentlemen and kept leaning on Dr Smith and me to get more patients into the rehabilitation centre. They wanted us to go out and canvass the hospitals. I did not think it was my place to go out and canvass patients and I felt that Dr Smith was also uncomfortable in this situation.

I next had a visit from a Dr Hayes, who was with the Department of Mental Health in Kentucky. He told me there was a Dr Burke working within his system. I told him I had known Dr Burke in Ireland and asked him to tell him to look me up. The following day I had a phone call from Dr Fintan Burke, whom I had not seen in over ten years.

He was living in a place called Hopkinsville, Kentucky, and said he would come to Louisville to visit me. We went out to eat with him the following week and he suggested that I should go and work with the state and that he could give me a job in Hopkinsville. He could pay me considerably more salary, together with free housing. My furnished apartment in Louisville was very expensive and this offer was too good to miss at the time.

I could get a temporary licence in the State of Kentucky until such time as I became a citizen and could then have a permanent licence. Everything pointed to Hopkinsville. However, the hospital was old and not in the same class as the rehabilitation centre. I would be in charge of the acute patients and acute treatment in Western State Mental Hospital. I was also given a supervisory position as Consultant in Physical Medicine and Rehab in the department to oversee rehabilitation in all Departments of Mental Health in Kentucky.

During this time Betty was making her way back from England and sailed into New York, where she caught a train for Kentucky. I met her in Louisville. I had to wait until August until the position was available with the State. Meanwhile, Betty and I explored Louisville, Fort Knox and the surrounding countryside, which looks beautiful in summer.

When everything was ready I resigned from the centre in Louisville and on 1 September started to work at Hopkinsville.

Being landlocked as we were in Kentucky, the existence was a bit dull. Many of the doctors were Cuban refugees and kept to themselves. The only people we got to know well were Dr Burke and his wife, as well as a doctor from Canada and his wife, who were also unhappy in Hopkinsville. However, I had to stay in one place for two years before I could take out citizenship, and Hopkinsville was where it was to be.

Our neighbours were from Cuba. The doctor was a refugee and one of his children had a birth defect in her hand. She was being looked after by a hand specialist in Louisville. It suited him to remain in Hopkinsville while his daughter had plastic surgery on her hand. We were never short of company and I always had someone to cover for me if we wanted to take trips to Nashville, Louisville or Frankfurt. In Nashville there were some very good restaurants. It was a long drive but we now had a good car, a Volkswagen Fastback which I had bought in Louisville.

During this period Japanese cars were beginning to get popular and I went to Clarksville to look at a new Toyota called a Crown. I just went in to look but when I sat in it the comfort was unbelievable. The price was even cheaper than the Volkswagen I was driving, which did not have air-conditioning, a radio or anything. They had four cars in the showroom but they were not selling because nobody knew anything about Japanese cars.

We decided that we needed a second car anyway and we bought it, little knowing it was going to be my door to my first Mercedes Benz.

Shortly after that I discovered that the state covered and gave time off for educational meetings. I headed for the annual Congress of Physical Medicine and Rehabilitation in Miami. During that visit I found that there really were no good jobs in rehabilitation even yet. I decided to stay on with the state until I could become a naturalized citizen.

In September 1968 I became a citizen of the United States in Paducah, Kentucky.

I awoke one night in October to find I had a bleeding ulcer. I was looked after in Madison Hospital in Kentucky, where I had surgery, after which I lost about 30 pounds. Kentucky was now a dead end. I was a citizen, I had a Kentucky licence passed by examination and there was no further reason to stay there.

My neighbour, Dr Loira, was also leaving as he had been appointed to a position in Puerto Rico. He had a good future as a general practitioner there.

I anticipated that Dr Burke would not remain in Hopkinsville much longer as the politics in the Mental Health Department were changing and he would probably be promoted to Louisville.

After looking through the journals, I sent some applications to the Veterans Administration, where all I needed was one licence in the United States to be legally employed. The Chief Medical Officer in Washington, DC, replied, recommending a position in Charleston, South Carolina. The Veterans hospital there had recently opened. He gave me details on how to apply. Within two weeks I was invited to come to Charleston for an interview as Chief of the Department in the new Veterans hospital. This was early in August and I decided to go immediately. I made the appointment to be interviewed and to see the hospital.

About that time there was a hurricane out in the Gulf of Mexico, called Camille. It came ashore and devastated the coastline of Mississippi. Gulfport was badly hit as well as Mobile, Alabama, then the hurricane moved inland, hitting Virginia and West Virginia. I had not anticipated that the hurricane would affect Kentucky but Betty and I took off and drove to Charleston and as it happened we went through the wake of the hurricane. We hit very high winds, torrential rains, thunder and lightning. It took us two days to get to South Carolina.

We were very impressed by Charleston, which is a beautiful city. The following morning we arrived at the Veterans Administration hospital, to find that some of the refugees from

Biloxi, Mississippi, had been transferred there. They had called to try and cancel my trip but I had already left Kentucky.

The interview went well and I found the staff to be very friendly. I met the Chief of Staff and the Administrator who were obviously anxious to have me come and join the staff. The physiatrist from the university, which was next door to the hospital, was too busy to run the department in the hospital. I left, promising to be back in two weeks. Our trip back to Kentucky was uneventful. Dr Burke was disappointed that I was leaving but he understood that there was not much future for my specialty in the State Mental Health Department.

Everything was shipped by Mayflower and the small stuff we packed into the two cars. I had a tow bar made that was attached to the Volkswagen, deciding to tow that with the Toyota Crown. The Crown had a six-cylinder engine and was quite powerful. It was one of the first Toyota cars in the country and I did not know that I was condemning it to a sad end.

We took the route through Nashville into Knoxville and on to Columbia, South Carolina, and from there to Charleston. It was hilly country but the car never flinched and we made excellent time, with one stop in Ashville. Superhighways had not been completed at that time so some of the trip was hard climbing and on very narrow roads. We had arranged to stay in an apartment house in north Charleston and we arrived on the second day.

After a few days getting oriented, I presented myself to the Veterans Administration and took over the department. It was well manned, with a good staff, physical and occupational therapists and even a speech therapy department. It was a beautiful hospital, with a complete library and the latest in equipment.

Our apartment was pleasant and we had very nice neighbours, with whom we became friendly. We found out through them that it would be nicer to live outside the city on the Isle of Palms, north of Charleston. We answered some advertisements for rental apartments on the island and we were interviewed by a Captain Wallerstedt, who presented us with a very exact contract to rent one of his houses. We decided to take it and arranged to move.

The Captain seemed a very stern gentleman but as it turned out he was a very kind man, friendly and amusing. We have been friendly ever since and keep in constant touch. We did not have access to the garage in the rental house because the Captain was keeping his sailboat in there. The weather was lovely so we were quite happy to park outside.

The drive into Charleston every day was enjoyable. The sea was on the left side with the inland waterway on the right. The traffic was never heavy and crossing the enormous bridge across the Cooper River at Mount Pleasant brought me right into the hospital.

After about six weeks the Toyota began to make strange noises and developed a knock in the engine. I took it to the local dealer, who kept it for two days and then informed me the car had ruined the front bearing, which had split in two. A main bearing in the engine was serious and expensive damage. As the car was out of warranty, this was going to cost at least $2,000, probably nearly as much as the car was worth.

I priced new cars but could not get a good price for the Toyota as dealers thought it would be difficult to sell. I then saw an advertisement for Mercedes Benz in a new agency outside Charleston. The car we could afford was a 220 gasoline Mercedes Benz, with no trimmings, no radio but with air-conditioner. I was surprised at the trade-in for the Toyota. It was twice as much as I could get anywhere else. I didn't deal then but went away and then came back. I finally got an excellent deal, left the Toyota and took away the Mercedes. Nobody had caught the problem in the front main bearing in the Toyota. They were dealers and it was their business to find it and not for me to show it to them.

When I arrived back with the Mercedes in the Isle of Palms, the Captain, whom we now called Stig, was so ashamed that we had no garage to put it in that he took his sailboat out and brought it to his own home and sold it. We now had a garage for our new car.

I brought the car back to the dealer to have its first 1,000 miles service and saw my old Toyota still sitting in their garage with the hood up and the engine out.

The bearing had been discovered and they found that they could not replace it. They ended up having to send to Japan for another one. The salesman told me about this and of course I was very surprised and told him I did not know anything about cars and was sorry that he seemed to be stuck with a dud. I told him he was the car specialist and I was just a customer. He took this very well and was always friendly when I went back. It was at least four months before the car was taken away and I felt very relieved that it was not there looking at me every time I brought back the Mercedes for service. The Volkswagen was sufficient for Betty, who only used it around the island for shopping and the occasional trip to Charleston. Unfortunately, on one of these trips she was rear-ended and the car was out of action for two weeks.

During the absence of the Volkswagen, Betty discovered that she could get a bus into Charleston and back and do shopping that way. We then decided to sell the Volkswagen to lighten our finances. We sold it to a naval cadet, who was very pleased with it. We bought two bicycles and we were able to cycle on the beach and Betty could cycle to the grocery store. Living on the Isle of Palms was very enjoyable.

After Stig had sold his sailboat, he decided to buy another one because the one he had sold was small and had no cabin. He bought a full-size sailboat with cabin which he called the *Sonata*. He spent most of his time getting it shipshape and when it was ready we had many pleasant sails with him.

I became acquainted with the politics of the Veterans Administration and discovered that my appointment to the department had been made in Washington and this had not gone down well with the local staff. Now I knew why such a fuss was made of my first visit and the attempt made to head off my interview. Apparently somebody else had been lined up for the position but they were not ready to come on short notice as I was.

Pressure was put on me to give up some of the space I had in my department. The occupational therapy department was next door to neurosurgery and that needed to expand. I resisted as long as I could but had to give in eventually and surrender some of my space. When that happened the chief of occupational therapy became huffed and accused me of not standing up for the department and she resigned. Next, some of the office space used by the physical therapists was commandeered and I had a very unhappy PT department as well as the OTs. Next I was asked to spend some time in the admissions department as my department was not very busy. This I refused to do and I found pressure being applied from all directions. After lunch the Administrator would come to my office to see if I was back from lunch on the dot. Sometimes he would be in the department when I came in in the morning, so I knew that I was an unwelcome member of the staff.

It was then suggested that I should work in the university and only part time in the VA hospital. Dr Mims in the university had neither the space nor the money to employ me. I decided then to start looking further afield and maybe move out of state.

On checking some of the journals for jobs, there was one in Jacksonville, Florida. I had to have a Florida licence, however, so I took the examination and passed. I then resigned from the Veterans hospital and took the job in the rehabilitation centre which was to be opened in Jacksonville, Florida.

The Jacksonville people would move me and help to finance furniture. In 1970 we moved to Florida and I started working in the new centre. We rented an apartment in Baymeadows Road, which was south of the city.

The official opening of the new centre was to be attended by Dr Howard Rusk of New York, whom I knew. The ceremony was very impressive and I met the local politicians, Dr Rusk and the doctors whose idea this rehabilitation centre was. There were no patients in the centre as yet and I had no idea of what they were going to do to fill beds. However, we had a nice apartment, new furniture, a decent car and everything was looking good. Our apartment building was new, at that time out in the country, and we were among the first occupants.

I was made a member of the Medical Society and I joined the Florida Medical Association. I applied for membership of all the hospitals in Jacksonville and was accepted by them all as I was the first and only physiatrist in Jacksonville. Each month the medical society met in the Hilton Hotel, and the various hospitals had their meetings on the same night. I addressed the meetings of the various hospitals and gave each a dissertation on what rehabilitation medicine was and what a physiatrist did and how I could help them. I told them there were beds available in the rehabilitation centre and this I thought was as far as I needed to go.

It transpired, however, that the members of the board of the centre thought that I should be doing more. They suggested that I should go to the hospitals where I had privileges and meet the staff in the mornings and generally canvass for patients and ask for consultations.

I had grown up in a different setting for medical practice and where I came from in Ireland and England canvassing was not considered to be an ethical approach to improving one's standing in the local community. I informed the board that this was what I thought, but some of the doctors told me that this was how they had built their practices and that this was the way it was done in America.

My reticence did not go down well but the pressure was kept on that this rehabilitation centre had to be occupied or else we would all go down with it. I was advised to visit other physiatrists in the state and to have their opinion about what I should do. The nearest physiatrist attached to the only hospital was in Orlando, which was then a very small town. He said he was looking for an assistant but that most of his practice was electromyography and the 'hands-on' rehabilitation practice was still in its infancy, even in Orlando.

Next I went to Tampa, Clearwater and St Petersburg and interviewed physiatrists there. None of them were writing prescriptions for physical therapy. Apparently, electromyography was where the money was. Now I look back and understand why Dr MacLean and I had been frozen out of electromyography at Yale. It was where the quick money was and where the jobs were.

I had seen an advertisement in the *Florida Medical Journal* looking for doctors in a place called New Port Richey. The advertisement had been placed by two doctors, a Dr Clark and a Dr Chovnick.

While in Clearwater I telephoned them and they told me to come up and see them. Before doing this I again visited the Clearwater physiatrist and he told me he was going to retire and would turn over his practice to me if I would agree to pay him off out of my takings. I counted that one out.

The two doctors in New Port Richey had charge of a new hospital which had just been opened and they received me with open arms. They were both surgeons but they needed more patients. They needed general practitioners to feed them. They would give me a free office and free staff if I joined their group. I would have all the amenities and have a complete take of all the patients I saw in my own office. I could not possibly turn this down.

I returned to Jacksonville, gave notice and Betty and I were once again moving. This time across Florida to New Port Richey on the Gulf.

15

Private Practice – Florida

The Clark Clinic was situated next to the Community Hospital in New Port Richey. The hospital was new, with 150 beds and plans were to expand to 300 beds. The clinic had a large waiting room with about eight examination rooms. Dr Clark and Dr Chovnick owned this. There were three doctors already on the staff and I was to be the fourth. We were later joined by four other doctors.

My practice flourished from the beginning. The office was fully staffed by secretaries and was run by a lady who had worked with Dr Clark for years and she oversaw all the office employees. At the end of the day I was handed the complete income from all patients I had seen for that day. There was no charge for rent or upkeep, everything was completely free.

Betty and I rented a small house not far from the hospital and installed our belongings. It was just another small Florida house in a small Florida street. It was adequate and everything was looked after by the landlord and his wife, who became my patients. There was a one-car garage in which we kept the Mercedes, and the Toyota Corolla station wagon we kept in the driveway.

The hospital emergency room was run by a staff who did nothing else. The patients were admitted to whichever doctor or doctors were on call for the day. On coming into the hospital the following morning, we were handed a list of admissions with diagnoses and all the paperwork already done.

Any patients that I admitted from the office were admitted directly without ado. The paperwork was completed in the office before the patient was even ready to go to the hospital, which was within 20 yards from my office.

My admission to the hospital staff was a formality. I was interviewed by the hospital Administrator, Andy Oravac, and the Chief of Staff, who was Dr Clark. The Assistant Chief of Staff was Dr Chovnick. Within two weeks I had ten patients in the hospital. The practice did so well because no other doctors in town were taking new patients. I was the twelfth doctor on the staff of Community Hospital.

My income was limited only by the amount of work I could do. The surgery consultations were adequate and if Doctors Clark or Chovnick were not available there was a surgeon across the street in the Richey Clinic. This clinic had stopped taking patients but their surgeon was willing to accept patients for surgery in Community.

In the hospital there was an active physical therapy department and I envisaged a busy physical medicine practice. This did not transpire, however, as the doctors on the staff knew nothing about rehabilitation medicine. Dr Clark advised me to canvass for patients and the Administrator agreed. To encourage me, the Administrator augmented my income by paying me a salary which was generous and kept me from getting depressed about the rehabilitation side of the practice.

General practice was booming, however, and I rapidly got back into the knowledge of cardiac and pulmonary diseases. The nursing staff of the intensive care unit were very knowledgeable and ready to give advice whenever I had a problem. I knew nothing about electrocardiography and had to put in an intensive course of study because nobody else on the staff knew any more than I did.

Very soon other doctors came to town and opened their offices and it was not long before the hospital was running at full capacity. After about six months a meeting was held in the office and it was decided by Dr Clark and Dr Chovnick that the newcomers should now begin to pay rent and contribute to the upkeep of the office staff. Some of us were not very happy with the way the office was being run and started looking out for our own office space.

I found a very nice office in Holiday, about 3 miles from New

Port Richey and Tarpon Springs. I rented this and we made plans to move there. One of the staff in Dr Clark's office asked to come with me. Betty volunteered to run the office as she had wide experience in legal and banking work. I told Jean from Dr Clark's office that she could come with me as she knew how to run a doctor's office inside out. She had worked in Tarpon Springs hospital and doctors' offices for years. She was a blessing and a wonderful lady to have working for me. Her loyalty was exceptional. Betty and she got on very well together and became close friends, and her husband was very helpful doing office repairs etc. We realized that we had made a good move and it could not go wrong.

I got in touch with a young attorney in Tampa, who advised that we should incorporate the practice and helped us set the whole thing up. He has been our attorney until this day.

The office was in excellent condition. It was over 2,000 square feet. It had been run by an osteopathic doctor who had left town. All we needed was to get furniture and some seats for the large waiting room. The seats were supplied free by a local funeral parlour and they said we could have them as long as we needed them. Betty said she was glad the patients did not know on whose seats they were sitting. Parking was adequate and the street was quiet but still very near the busy main highway, Highway 19, between New Port Richey, Clearwater, Tampa and St Petersburg.

In about two months we were ready to build a house, which we did on Madison Street, close to the hospital. It was a quiet little street in those days and we had the house built to our own specifications by a very helpful builder.

Our new neighbours were very friendly. On one side we had an Irish lady with an American husband who kept to themselves. On the north side there was a pleasant couple with two daughters and they were also very quiet. It was sad that the father of the children had had kidney surgery and many problems, from which he died over a year later.

The practice continued to flourish and in six months I sold the Toyota station wagon to our secretary, Jean, and bought a Nissan 240Z.

I became an active member of the Pasco County Medical

Society and a year later was elected as Secretary/Treasurer. This post I retained until I was elected as President in 1980.

Madison Street had been a quiet street when we built our house, with no houses on the opposite side. In six months houses were built on the far side and it was decided to build a bridge at the end of the street, which had been a dead end on the river. It was now difficult for me to get out in the mornings as I had to back out from the driveway into the traffic. After two years it was apparent that we would have to get a bigger house. Jean, our secretary, started looking around and found us a very nice house on the water in the bay at Port Richey and there was a boat that went with it. We bought it and, although it needed some repair, we considered it to be worth it.

I applied for staff membership in Tarpon Springs hospital and was accepted. I also was appointed Medical Director in the only nursing home in town as no other doctor wanted to follow patients there. Doctors on the staff found it very convenient to ask me to look after their patients while in the nursing home, which I did. Eventually there were four other nursing homes built in the area and I looked after most of the patients in them and could visit them once a week. Unfortunately, Medicare changed the rules and only paid for one medical visit per month. I continued to see my patients more frequently and at the request of the nursing staff. However, it became uneconomical to follow patients under these circumstances. I then had to refuse to accept patients in the nursing homes.

In 1974 I took a day off in the middle of the week to attend a medical meeting in Tampa, so the office was not open on that day. On the way home I dropped by the office to check if there were any patients needing to be seen. I found police cars, photographers, the press and a general furore in the parking lot. There was a large hole in the waiting room wall and the window had been demolished. Apparently an elderly gentleman turned into our parking lot and couldn't stop. He drove through the waiting room wall, nearly hitting the secretary, who had been sitting behind the reception counter. Jean was in a state of shock and Betty had been sent for. A photograph of our office was in the local newspapers the following day. I am not sure if that brought us any more business but it was one way to advertise.

In the Tarpon Springs hospital there was a fairly active physical therapy department and I got a few consultations but never enough to be able to go into rehabilitation full-time.

In 1975 Community Hospital was taken over by the Hospital Corporation of America, who built a new four-storey wing and expanded the hospital to about 500 beds. The number of doctors on the staff now was increasing and I was elected Chief of the Department of Medicine.

New Port Richey was finally on the map and was expanding rapidly. The growth was so fast that it was decided to build a new hospital about 10 miles north in a suburb called Bayonet Point. This was also a three-storey hospital with about 250 beds. Most of the staff of Community Hospital were also accepted there.

There were subdivisions going up like mushrooms all over the area around New Port Richey. The population was increasing rapidly. Bayonet Point had been out in the country when the hospital was built but in two years it was also surrounded by private homes as retirees were pouring down from the north. It was one of the most rapidly growing areas in Florida in the 1970s and early 1980s.

About this time patient admissions to the hospital became very restricted and the length of time a patient stayed in the hospital was limited by the new system, which went under the name of DRGs (Diagnostic Related Groups). This meant that every diagnosis that could be imagined was limited to a certain length of time in hospital. Myocardial infarction was limited to about a ten-day stay at the most. Stroke was limited about the same and acute appendicitis was cut down to about three to five days, and so on and so forth. Regardless of how severe a patient's illness was, their stay in the hospital had to be justified after the DRG time had expired. Doctors were very frustrated at being accosted in the corridors of the hospital by secretaries, most of them 17 to 22 years of age, querying the length of time certain patients were in the hospital. They wanted to know when they would be discharged and what was the reason for their extended stays.

Prior to this if a patient did not want to go home for the weekend, they would be left in hospital. Sometimes the relatives were going to be away or had something organized and did not want their parents or children sent home until after the weekend. DRGs changed all this, and there was even a threat that if the patients were kept longer than the DRG time, the doctor would be charged by the hospital for the extra time because Blue Cross and Blue Shield and Medicare would not pay for it. It was about this time that payment for the nursing home visits were curtailed to one a month.

At this stage I was attending about five nursing homes as well as running the practice. I was running into problems at night, when nurses would call me for the slightest excuse and even have me come and see patients who were not actually registered with me at all but with some other doctor who refused to go to the nursing home.

I could not decide to stop attending nursing homes because I had so many patients of my own that I would be abandoning. Nobody else was going to look after them if I did not. It was a no-win situation.

I decided that I would sit for the Board examination in physical medicine and rehabilitation as it had been started up again. I had neglected to take this exam within the three years of finishing my residency at Yale, and the regulations made me ineligible if I had not taken it within this time.

Now it was opened up again upon the demise of the old specialty director in Rochester, Minnesota. A younger man had been appointed to bring the rules up to date. He sent an invitation to all eligible doctors, specialists in PM&R, inviting them to take the examination and become Board Certified.

In 1979 I took the examination, became Board Certified, and decided I would look around and see what was available in Florida in my specialty.

An attractive job came up in Jupiter, Florida, and I went to interview the doctor who was making the offer. He wanted a physiatrist full time in a pain clinic. I decided to get out of New Port Richey and get away from the nursing homes, DRGs and all the problems and take the job.

* * *

I put my practice up for sale and I got a lady doctor from India who had just started in New Port Richey. She offered to take the practice and buy the office. About this time some of the doctors on the staff in Community Hospital asked me if I would go forward as Chief of Staff. I had already burned my boats so I had to decline.

Before going to Jupiter I called my attorney and told him what I was doing. He advised me to be cautious and volunteered to come down to Jupiter to a meeting with Dr Shams and a company called McCanns (a namesake of my own) in order to set up a proper legal agreement, which had been proposed by the other party.

During the meeting it transpired that Dr Shams and the McCanns had intended that I should invest in the practice. My attorney said this was impossible and in no way could this be done. An agreement was arrived at eventually and I could go and practise without investing. Unfortunately, the salary I would get was much smaller without the investment. Boats being burned again, I decided to go along with it anyway, in the hope of getting some private practice as well. There was no objection to this.

I made an arrangement with a small motel to rent by the month and got a reduced rate. I would go home on the weekends.

The practice did not flourish at all. Dr Shams was a psychiatrist and not very conversant with pain problems as I understood them, but we continued and I hoped that things would pick up. I applied for privileges in the hospital nearby. Although Dr Shams was on the staff, my privileges were refused. The staff was already overloaded. I applied to all the hospitals in the area but none of them were taking new doctors at that time.

I stuck it out in Jupiter for six months but fortunately I had not cut myself off from New Port Richey. We still had our house and Betty was living there, so I decided to go back and open an office 10 miles north of my old one to try to rebuild a practice. Despite the entreaties of the nursing homes, I refused to get back into that branch of medicine. Many of my old patients who lived near my new office came back. A third that lived in the area close to my old office I could not take back because it would have been a threat to the doctor who had taken my first practice.

Going back anywhere never works, so I began to look for positions out of state in my specialty. In May 1983 I got a letter from an old friend, a doctor who had been a part-time professor at Yale. He was a physiatrist in Washington, DC, at the VA Hospital. He was about to resign and he wanted to have a say in the appointment of whoever succeeded him. This was a godsend as the second practice was not getting off the ground.

I went to Washington at the expense of the Veterans Administration and met Dr Kaminitz and was interviewed by the Administrator, Chief of Staff, Chief of Surgery and the chiefs of all the departments. Dr Kaminitz took me to his home for dinner, cooked by his charming French wife.

Dr Kaminitz had no doubt that I would get the appointment, so I returned to New Port Richey and within a week I had a telephone call to say I was appointed and I would start on 1 July 1983.

I turned my second practice over to Dr Milam, a friend whom I had known for some five years, as he had decided to open his own practice. Unfortunately, he was killed in an air crash ten years later.

Betty and I went to Washington and rented a car to look around. We found a very nice furnished apartment in Alexandria, Virginia, which was run by a California firm and had a very reasonable rent, even for Washington, DC.

The salary was excellent, but only when I had moved and lived in Washington did I find out it was not excessive but adequate.

16

Washington, DC

I left Betty in Florida to sell our house in Port Richey. We had put on a second floor and it was now quite a big house. We had done this in 1979 and it was finished shortly after I had passed the Board examination. The examination had paid off in that I got the job in Washington, DC, for which a Board certification was a prerequisite.

On 1 July 1983 I took over the Department of Physical Medicine and Rehabilitation at the Veterans Administration Hospital. The department was very large, with a staff of 20, including physical, occupational and recreational therapists. It had a very large swimming pool and even a department where patients were taught carpentry, engineering, leather work, book binding etc., much of which was new to me. My administrative assistant was Phylis DiLullo.

There were two other doctors in the department, neither of whom was Board certified, but Dr Chacko was eligible and was taking the exam the following year. Another doctor, an Italian, was marking time in the department, having headed the vascular surgery section in the VA head office for some years. His position had been eliminated, however, and the job in the VA physical medicine department had been made for him. He came in at 11.00 a.m. and left at 3.00 p.m. He was paid full salary for this and he knew absolutely nothing about rehabilitation medicine and was unwilling to learn.

I volunteered to help him get his boards if he would come in and work a full day and learn how to do electromyography and nerve conduction studies, and go and take a refresher course. He was highly insulted with these suggestions and left. It was good for the department because there was less of a drag on the financial resources as the budget was very tightly controlled.

The department was closely associated with George Washington University and Georgetown University. I was expected to apply for staff membership on both those hospitals. I applied and was duly accepted. I also applied for staff privileges in the Howard University, but my letter was not answered.

Dr Kaminitz continued to be helpful in the department and he visited and gave lectures once a week.

Meanwhile Betty was in New Port Richey and our house was on the market. Finally, we sold it at a loss. We then needed an apartment in Washington, and the Italian doctor, with whom I was still friendly at this stage, suggested the Irene Apartments. I looked at an apartment there and, although it was very big, I decided to take it. The carpeting came with it but when I was leaving I found that if the next tenant did not want the carpet I would have to pay to have it taken out and the baseboards reset to their original setting.

The apartment was very dark and gloomy and Betty was very unhappy in it. We started looking again and got a very nice one on the eighteenth floor of The Promenade, an apartment building overlooking the Beltway at Pooks Hill. We were much more comfortable and happier there.

In the hospital I had certainly been fortunate to inherit Dr Kaminitz's administrative assistant, Phylis DiLullo. She had been working for the Veterans Administration in other departments and knew the regulations and the rules inside out and back to front. She was of inestimable value and understood all the angles in the bureaucracy and never let me get into any jams.

She was a wonderful cook and loved a picnic. Each month I had to attend meetings in other Veterans Administration hospitals outside Washington. Phylis would make all the arrangements and after the meeting we would have a picnic. She brought all the food, drinks, table linen, everything. I had never had picnics like that either before or since. Dr Kaminitz frequently came along with us.

Phylis retired in 1985 and the department was never the same again. There was a residential programme in George Washington University for rehabilitation medicine residents and they rotated through the department, making the work much easier. Dr Chacko sat for her Boards and passed them first time.

After we finally sold our house in Florida, we decided we would not give up our Florida residency. We bought a small patio home in St Augustine, which was the most appealing place to live in Florida. It was north and nearest to Washington. Although it was an 800-mile trip, we could commute up and down. Later we discovered the auto train which went from Sanford, Florida, to Washington.

Betty was not compelled to stay in Washington around the year and she could fly back and forth to Florida and would meet me at the airport in Jacksonville when I flew down on some weekends. There was a restaurant in our apartment building in Pooks Hill and plenty of restaurants in Washington, so when I was on my own I could fend for myself.

In 1987 I decided I should be on the lookout for some position in Florida that would be closer to home and I saw an advertisement for doctors in the prison system in Florida. They were looking for internists and family practitioners. By now I would have had five years in the Veterans Administration, having spent time in Charleston, SC, for which I would get credit. This meant I could now retire with many benefits including the Federal Blue Cross & Blue Shield health insurance and a small pension if I timed it properly.

I applied for a job with the Department of Corrections in Florida. I was interviewed and obtained a position in Daytona Beach in the Tomoka Prison. I resigned from the VA and decided to head back to Florida.

17

Prison Doctor

Having resigned from the Veterans Administration, I could not just walk away. Before I could get my pension, sickness insurance, life insurance and various other benefits, I had to visit every department in the hospital to get a clearance that I had no outstanding records, debts or unfinished business of any kind. This meant waiting around until the appropriate person became available to sign my personnel chart and confirm that I was at liberty to leave.

On my last day I had a nice send-off party in a restaurant downtown, with presentations and souvenirs etc. There were photographs taken and the number of people attending from the department and from the hospital, surprised me. The medical staff gave me a party also and by and large I found I was more popular than I had thought.

Getting out of our apartment was another problem. We were on the eighteenth floor and as far from the elevators as it was possible to get, so it was a long process. The temperature that day was up in the nineties, which didn't help. When we had the apartment finally emptied, we moved to a motel and let the furniture go ahead. We had both cars and packed them with our personal goods and said farewell to Washington.

We spent the first night in North Carolina. Betty was driving the Maxima with the U-Haul roof-rack on top and I drove the Mercedes. We finally reached St Augustine on the second day, very glad to be back permanently in Florida.

* * *

The initiation into the prison system took about a week. This included being photographed, fingerprinted and instructed in the ways of the prison and the prisoners. There were other employees being initiated at the same time so we were all gathered in a classroom and addressed by various members of the staff including the Superintendent, warders, psychologists and various other staff whose job it was to keep inmates (as they were called) within the limits of the prison and under control.

We were instructed as to the deviousness of inmates, their methods of manipulation of staff and avoidance of work and obtaining privileges. In general we were being convinced that inmates were scoundrels, not to be trusted, not to be believed and not to be given an inch under any circumstances. We were brought on a tour of the prison and shown the security systems, the double perimeter with razor wire on top and towers at all corners. On top of each tower was at least one guard with rifle and shotgun.

About this time there was an ongoing legal battle in Florida. The inmates, represented by two lifers, sued the government for better conditions for inmates and improved medical treatment. They wanted access to medical specialists and hospitals as frequently as necessary. The case had been in progress for about three years and continued for nearly another three. It was finally settled much to the advantage of the inmates. While it was going on, there were frequent visits to all the Florida prisons by teams of inspectors, who checked that the inmates were being well treated and receiving the best of medical attention. I found that this was why I and other doctors were being employed at that time. There were now two doctors in the Tomoka prison where there had been one previously. All the prisons where there had been part-time doctors were now to have full-time doctors, with nursing and ancillary staff.

When I finally got to work I found that most of the inmates were quite healthy but they all wanted to get to the sickbay to see the new doctors to find out how they could manipulate them and get benefits.

The hospital was well equipped, with a comprehensive pharmacy.

The patients were a mixed lot, with some quite respectable

ones, businessmen, retirees, burglars, murderers and many serving time for having been caught with drugs. There were child molesters, wife beaters, thieves, especially car thieves, conmen and what have you.

The inmates were very ready to talk about their sentences, and their crimes – of which they were all innocent – and all could give very convincing stories as to how they had been framed. Only once did I meet an inmate who said that he had committed a crime and that he was justifiably confined.

This one exception was a man with whom, oddly enough, I got very friendly. He was hated by the guards and feared by other prisoners. He was called 'Animal'. The first time I met Animal he came to the hospital with a very acute abdominal pain. He was antagonistic, but because of his severe pain he had no alternative but to come and be examined. He looked like Kojak and shaved his head, probably every day. On examination of his abdomen he had scars and all the evidence of having been in accidents or fights. He had scars on his arms and his legs, with many tattoos, and looked a very ferocious man. He was obviously suffering from cholecystitis or his gall bladder was inflamed, and he had to go to hospital. I got him transferred to the hospital in Daytona and the following day, more out of curiosity than an attempt to be friendly, I visited him.

He had had surgery immediately upon admission and a cholecystectomy performed, but he was still in considerable pain. He recognized me and asked me for a cigarette. I told him I didn't have any and that I didn't smoke. The guards refused to give him any cigarettes. There was a guard sitting with him night and day, and when Animal wasn't going to the bathroom he was chained to the bed. He asked me if I could get him some cigarettes. I couldn't get any in the hospital so I went downtown Daytona, bought a carton and brought them back to him, with matches.

His disbelief and gratitude almost brought tears to my eyes. He had never apparently had any kindness like this from the time he was put in prison. He had been a motorcycle bandit, a very fierce man who had had fights with police. He had been shot by the police and he had shot a policeman. Even his knuckles were scarred from bare-knuckle fights. He had scars on his head and his face from fights and he had been told by the guards in the prison that they would be delighted to have an excuse to shoot him if he became violent. Because of this he was fairly peaceful during the time that I knew him. He told me he hated cops and the prison guards.

Animal's recovery was uneventful. He was well fed while he was in the hospital and was soon back in prison. I visited him frequently and he showed me his workshop, where he made leather goods of very high quality indeed. He also made wooden knick-knacks, which he was allowed to sell in a limited market. He asked me what he could make for me out of leather. Did I need a briefcase, this that and other things? I could think of nothing except a wallet, and then I remembered I needed a passport case. He made me one which was stamped and designed in three colours. I was very grateful and he had to slip it to me as I was not allowed to take it. Somehow he got it to my office, I don't know how. I never asked. He had printed the case with my name.

Whenever I was not busy I would visit Animal and he was very entertaining. He would not eat in the cafeteria and had his food brought to him. He had lackeys and other inmates who tended to him and looked after him. Generally he was a king in his own little kingdom. When we talked, he would get the other inmates out of earshot. He only needed to shout at them as though they were dogs and they cowed and moved away. He told me that if I had any problems with prisoners while I was there, or if anybody gave me a hard time to let him know. I never needed to get his help but it was comforting to know that as he was a friend of mine I was probably safe from any attack or riots that might take place. He was certainly the most interesting inmate I met in my stay in Tomoka. It did not endear me with the guards that I was friendly with him and some of them told me I had been crazy to bring him cigarettes. As it turned out, it was one of the best things I could have done.

My job was made very easy by the fact that I had an excellent head nurse, who was also manager of the hospital. He was an ex-marine and had been a medic. He knew more about bacteriology and some lab procedures than I did. He was very helpful and became a great friend, and still is to this day.

After six months in Tomoka I heard that there was a vacancy for a doctor in a prison in Palatka, which was within easy driving distance from my home. I applied for a transfer and got it.

Palatka was a much smaller prison and the supervision of the inmates was much tighter. Even so, two escaped while I was there. Most of their crimes were of a minor nature compared to the inmates of Tomoka. Many of them were in Palatka awaiting discharge or parole, and they mostly worked every day on the roads or on projects in the county. Some worked on farms and some on building projects, some even worked on the building of a new golf course in Keystone Heights, the town in which the Superintendent lived. They were younger by and large than in Tomoka and less manipulative. They all, when they got sick, asked me to give them Dove soap, which was a great favourite.

Most of the African Americans wanted to be allowed to grow beards, claiming that they developed skin rashes from shaving with the safety razors and the resulting ingrowing facial hair. Most of them wanted to get shoes other than the prison boots, which they said caused blisters on their feet when they worked on the roads.

When I granted too many of these privileges the Superintendent became very irate and visited me and told me that these people were manipulating me, whereupon he began to manipulate me.

He asked me for prescriptions, mostly for mild pain medications, until one day he asked me to write a prescription for his son for a narcotic. He said his doctor usually gave him this but he wanted to save the office fee that he would have to pay the doctor.

Fortunately, I saw the red flag and informed him that I could not treat him or his family because I had no medical malpractice insurance for treating patients outside the prison. I also told him it would be malpractice to treat patients whom I had never seen and for conditions that I had not diagnosed. From that day on the Superintendent was distinctly unfriendly and, looking back on it, I realized that my days were numbered in the prison system.

There was an area director physician, who had his office in Gainesville, and he visited hospitals occasionally and had meetings every month. He had been in on my interview when I was employed and he certainly knew the prison system. In Tomoka when I attended his meetings, I brought my hospital manager with me and he really did most of the work, taking notes and keeping good records. When I went to Palatka I did not have that advantage because my manager was a young lady and she was not well versed in the procedures, records keeping and the cunning ways of inmates and those in charge of them. I later found out that this lady had the ear of the Superintendent and that she and a very attractive nurse visited frequently with him.

The inmates were mostly young dropouts from school and I advised many of them to attend the very good school in the prison and get their GED to finish their education. Many of them did, and made this their excuse for not going to work on the roads. The Superintendent visited me and protested that I was only supposed to give the inmates medical attention and not to advise on their education or other matters.

When I started to work for the prisons there was a clause in the contract that said physicians could be discharged for no reason. I do not know why that was there and I had already agreed to work for the system when I found this out. The Superintendent put this clause to good use on the last day of June 1988. When I arrived at the gate to go through to my office I was told that I could no longer come into the prison and that the Superintendent had given orders that I was to be discharged. There was no reason given; there was no reason needed. So I emptied my office and left. When I asked the Superintendent the reason for my discharge, he said there was no reason, I was not entitled to one. He had apparently written me a letter to the effect that I was discharged but I did not receive it for six weeks. He said it must have been lost in the mail!

When I protested to my Regional Medical Director, he said he couldn't give a reason and that he didn't know. It was the Superintendent's privilege and there was nothing he could do about it. This was the answer I got all the way up to Tallahassee.

So ended my experience with the Florida penal system, or the Department of Corrections. In the following week I applied for unemployment benefits and was granted them on guaranteeing that I would immediately start searching for another job.

As usual, Betty did all the paperwork and was very helpful in getting us the unemployment benefits and searching the newspapers for positions. I had never looked in the newspapers for jobs, certainly not medical jobs for doctors, but surprisingly one was advertised paying $20,000 more a year than I was receiving in the prisons. I applied and had some interesting interviews and began my experience in a charity clinic in Madison County, Florida.

18

Postponing Retirement

In September 1988, after interviews, I was appointed Medical Director of the Tri-County Medical Center in Greenville, Florida. Greenville was in Madison County and the capital of Madison County is Madison City, where there is a hospital. The clinic had an office in a converted home on a side street in Madison. The clinic itself was in a mobile home on a piece of waste ground across from the hospital. The hospital had about 50 beds. In the mobile home (a double-wide) there were three examination rooms and various small offices. There were three nurses, a nurse practitioner and a practitioner's assistant. The manager who ran the whole operation lived in Tallahassee and worked out of the central office of the clinic in Greenville.

I was replacing a local surgeon who had been the director of the clinic but wished to resign. When I was appointed, an osteopathic physician resigned and went to practise in Pensacola. There was also a branch clinic in Perry, about 60 miles south.

The clinic was financed by the National Health Organization of Washington, DC.

There was a lot of rivalry between the local private doctors and the clinic, and when I arrived I was invited by the Administrator of the hospital to a staff meeting. As I had been invited without the approval of the staff, it was announced at the meeting that if I applied for privileges at the hospital I would not be approved. Rather than have it on my record that I was refused privileges in a hospital, I did not apply, and destroyed the application I had already filled out. The osteopathic doctor who had been in the clinic before me had had privileges in the hospital and he told me that there was much resentment when he was on call.

I ran morning clinics in Madison in the mobile home and did afternoon clinics in Greenville. The patients had a great variety of problems but one of the most prominent was overweight. There was not a day that I did not see at least five patients over 250 pounds and many over 300 pounds. Some were even up to 400 pounds. Most of them were women. There was quite a bit of gynaecology, pap tests and general examinations, varicose ulcers and pediatrics of all descriptions. Anything that was possible in the pediatric field, I saw.

The geriatric practice, with heart and lung problems, was quite large. Quite a lot of emphysema, asthma and bronchitis – everyone smoked.

I decided to stay in the local motel until I got somewhere to live, and I employed a local estate agent to find me a place. After the first morning touring homes, I should have fired him. The first place he showed me was a mobile home in a field with no steps leading up to the door, just a ladder. There was no running water and no possibility of having a telephone. The next home he showed me was still furnished. There was a refrigerator that had not been cleaned out and still had food in it with green mould, and rotten vegetables and meat.

Finally, I did rent a home 2 miles from downtown Madison which did have electricity and a telephone, but the cable TV did not reach that far. The former occupant was the owner and he rented it to us while he went to Orlando to open a restaurant. He was Chinese and the brother of one of the local physicians.

The house was down in the hollow of a field and when we tried to get a television antenna it was below the level of the surrounding hills. We had to put up an enormously high antenna to get even the Tallahassee stations. We then moved in, but one of the big problems was there was no driveway down to the house from the highway, just a gravel path. Whenever it rained, the gravel washed away and it was nearly impossible to drive up to the highway.

Not having privileges in the local hospital and having to send any acutely ill patients to Lake City, 70 miles away, my position in

Madison was not particularly attractive and I knew I should keep looking elsewhere to settle permanently.

We had kept our home in St Augustine, so on weekends whenever I was not on call we went home. It was a long trip on Highway 10 to Jacksonville and then down to St Augustine but it was a relief to get out of the house in the field.

There was only one place in Madison to get groceries when we first went there, and that was the Winn Dixie. The parking lot for some reason always had dead snakes all over the place whenever Betty went shopping there. She said it was like Africa all over again. The selection of food was dismal which explained the number of obese patients because there was not much other than fat meat and chicken. Before we left, the Food Lion opened a store at the other end of town, but we were already leaving by the time they arrived.

There was one restaurant in town and there was another one out on Highway 10 which catered to truckers and had quite good food.

Tallahassee was 55 miles away, so on the weekends that we did not go home we went there. Another escape was Valdosta, Georgia, which was about 40 miles to the north. There were some fairly good restaurants there.

Although this job paid well it was certainly not attractive and with the problems with the hospital constantly in the background I had to decide to leave.

A position became available in the Sunland Center in Gainesville and I applied to become Assistant Medical Director. I was interviewed and accepted. In July 1989 we moved out of Madison, stored the furniture and soon found a nice townhouse in Gainesville, not far from the Sunland Center. The centre is a very old establishment, consisting of separate chalets spread over a 50-acre park. Each chalet is called after a flower and run by an independent team. The patients are mostly retarded children and adults, and they are segregated more or less according to their disabilities. They have a personal staff night and day to look after them and they have excellent medical attention. There were then about ten doctors on the staff, each doctor having four or five chalets to look after. I was given five chalets to look after. The doctors attend each chalet every day and any acute condition is sent into the central clinic to be looked after. The medical attention is comprehensive and all diagnostic facilities are available. The Medical Director had recently been appointed and I anticipated filling the position of Assistant Medical Director but the position never transpired.

After serving as a staff physician there for six months I got an offer in rehabilitation medicine near Orlando, so I resigned from the Sunland Center and we moved to Orlando.

This clinic was run by a retired orthopaedic surgeon. It was strictly a personal injury clinic and all the patients had been in automobile or other accidents. Their care was being paid for by insurance companies and it was a semi-rehabilitation clinic. It was staffed by RNs and three doctors.

The retired surgeon had taken over the operation from another physician. My job was to see patients who had been sent to the clinic for evaluation after automobile or Workmen's Compensation accidents. When I examined the patients I then wrote the reports, which had to be sent to the insurance companies who had referred the patients. I dictated my reports and they were sent out to be typed. When the typed reports came back, I discovered they had been altered and the reports that I was signing were not the reports I had dictated. They had been modified by the doctor. I was naturally unhappy with this situation and resigned and left Orlando.

Just after leaving Orlando I had interviewed a Dr Lenhart in St Petersburg, Florida. His operation was well organized, he being German, and self-made. He had started out as a chiropractic physician and put himself through medical school, becoming a physiatrist and doing his residency in Emory University.

While I was deciding whether I would work with Dr Lenhart or not, I got a phone call from a Dr Feinstein in Miami Beach, who flew up in his own plane to St Augustine and flew Betty and me back. He showed us his practice in north Miami Beach and offered me half as much again as Dr Lenhart. He rented me a car to drive back to St Augustine. We were put up in a hotel in Fort Lauderdale for the night and wined and dined at his club. My final decision was to work in Miami Beach instead of St Petersburg. Dr Lenhart told me that if ever I changed my mind to go back and see him again.

The position in Miami Beach would be temporary. Dr Feinstein was an osteopathic physician who had a combination of personal injury from car accidents and Workmen's Compensation patients, together with some general practice. If I spent more than ten minutes with a patient in an examination room, the secretary came and knocked on the door to ask me if there was anything holding me up. Finally I tried to get one of the patients off a medication on which he was becoming dependent. The patient complained to the owner of the practice. We disagreed and I left on short notice.

I went back to St Augustine and spent Christmas there, having left Miami Beach in November 1990. I contacted Dr Lenhart in St Petersburg again, and went to join him in his practice early in 1991. We kept our home in St Augustine, and although the commute was about 200 miles one way, I did this on most weekends until 1994. We had found a small apartment in north St Petersburg which was adequate and not too far from my office.

Dr Lenhart had been running his practice with a physician's assistant and a husband-and-wife team of chiropractors. The male chiropractor left shortly after I arrived and also the physician's assistant. Dr Lenhart and Dr Dunn, a lady chiropractor, and I, then continued the practice. After Dr Dunn and I had taken histories and done physical examinations, Dr Lenhart then examined the patient and ordered X-rays, tests etc. He then followed the patients for the rest of their time attending the clinic.

Dr Lenhart taught me how to do electromyography and nerve conduction studies, which was very useful. This filled in the gap which had remained since my days at Yale. He was an excellent teacher, showing me everything once and then telling me, 'Now, you do it.' I had no alternative but to get back to my books and learn. Dr Lenhart never pulled his punches and if anything happened of which he did not approve he said it right out. He could find and see immediately a flaw in the history or a physical examination and we became very punctilious regarding the details of histories, physicals and reporting. Soon the practice was running smoothly and Dr Lenhart left me on my own quite frequently and soon depended upon me to run it when he wasn't there.

In February 1992 during a routine check-up in Mayo Clinic, Betty was discovered to be suffering from cancer of the breast. I took time off and her surgeon recommended a mastectomy immediately. She was moved over to the care of Dr W. Maples in the Oncology Department at Mayo. She was placed on Tamoxifen after she had recovered from the surgery, and continued to be closely watched and followed up at regular intervals.

When she had recovered, we got back into our routine of going to St Augustine on weekends and going back to St Petersburg early on Monday mornings.

After I had left Orlando we had decided to leave our small house on St Augustine beach and build a larger house in Marsh Creek, a golf course community in St Augustine. Our house looked out onto the golf course and it was very comfortable. We lived there until we sold it in 1996 to move to Ocala, Florida.

The practice in St Petersburg continued uneventfully until 1993 when Dr Lenhart began to practise hair transplants, and more of the personal injury practice fell to me and Dr Dunn.

For some unknown reason the number of patients seeking care for personal injuries began to decrease, although the hair transplant part of the practice was flourishing.

In October 1994 Dr Lenhart came to me and told me the practice was going down and that there was not enough business to support two doctors and he would have to let me go. On 31

October 1994 I did my last day's work in St Petersburg. Betty and I packed and moved back to St Augustine.

I was now 71 years of age and I decided that I would have to retire as I did not think anyone would want to employ a doctor of my age.

I began to get busy with my library and to read the books that I had been promising myself I would eventually read, including Shakespeare and some of the classics. I read Homer's *Odyssey* and then started on the *Iliad* which was heavy going. The *Odyssey*, however, inspired the title of this book.

During the previous year when Dr Lenhart became interested in the hair transplant business I had instinctively felt that my position was insecure. At that time I answered an advertisement in the *Florida Medical Journal* for a position in a Bariatric Clinic in Ocala, Florida. Ocala is about halfway between St Petersburg and St Augustine. I received a phone call from the owner of the clinic, a Mr Bill Provost. He said that I was a bit late as he had already employed someone, but he took all the information I gave him and said he would keep me in mind in case the doctor he had employed did not work out.

Lo and behold in April 1995 I had a phone call from Bill. He asked if I was still interested in joining his weight reduction clinic. I could not believe my good fortune and I assured him I was still interested and how soon could I come? He said, 'Immediately.' Two days later I visited him in Ocala in a beautiful clinic, two buildings and windows everywhere. There was lots of room and real daylight in every part of it. Somewhat different from Dr Lenhart's clinic, where it was dark, gloomy and all artificially lighted.

Betty came with me and we talked for a long time with Bill in his clinic. We got on very well together. I made an arrangement with a local Holiday Inn that I could spend three days a week there at a reduced rate. I would be working a 20-hour week with Bill and be free on Thursday afternoon through Sunday. I would only be working Monday through Thursday morning. It was not a tiring commute from St Augustine to Ocala. I had to go through the Ocala National Forest and it was a pleasant drive.

We decided, however, that we would buy a home in Ocala and

sell the St Augustine house. We did this and moved to Ocala in January 1996. We built a smaller house in Ocala, where we have been ever since.

The practice is booming and Bill is a wonderful man to work for. He is a layman who owns the clinic, but he has to have a doctor to run it and I was elected.

My children are both married. My son has three children and my daughter has three. They are well and my son is living in Southern Ireland and my daughter is in Northern Ireland. We have friendly communication and I am sure this book will be revealing to them both.

Betty continues well, although she had some recurrences, for which she is, at the time of writing, having chemotherapy treatments. She has been well looked after at the Mayo Clinic and no stone is left unturned to keep her comfortable and well.

We have no plans for further travel or change of status. However, with my record, who knows what may come next?